Inspirational

Cryptograms

Vol. 4

Large print

Edie Gaines

Printed by: CreateSpace
7290 B. Investment Drive
Charleston, SC 29418

To order the book, go to:
www.createspace.com/4074399

Manufactured in the United States of America
Printed on 30% recycled paper.

ISBN – 10: 148123448X
ISBN-13: 978-1481234481(CreateSpace-Assigned)

DEDICATION

To my friend
Bruce Coyle,
Thank you
for all the
inspiring emails,
darling!

Love you!

Other cryptogram books by Edie:

Inspirational Cryptograms
It is available at: **www.createspace.com/3564509**

Inspirational Cryptograms Vol. 2
It is available at: **www.createspace.com/3666400**

Inspirational Cryptograms Vol. 3
It is available at: **www.createspace.com/4054734**

The Inspirational Cryptograms series is a collection of inspiring and motivational quotes. You'll find thought provoking and humorous quotes about life, in general, from some famous and not so famous people.

Political Cryptograms of the 60's & 70's
      This book is intended to appeal to those with an historical or political interest. It is a collection of quotes and facts from those Presidential campaigns, which were watersheds in American history, as well as facts and quotes from other key figures. It is available at: **www.createspace.com/3558992**

All books are done in large print.

TABLE OF CONTENTS

Introduction   vi

Hints to solve cryptograms   vii

Puzzles   1

Clues:

    #1   111

    #2   116

Solutions   121

INTRODUCTION

Cryptograms are a great exercise for the mind. Both pattern recognition and linear thought are necessary in code breaking. This is an excellent exercise to train the mind to think using both halves of the brain.

Inspirational Cryptograms, Vol. 4, as with previous volumes in the series, is a collection of inspiring and motivational quotes. You'll find some thought provoking and humorous quotes about life, in general, for your decoding pleasure.

The print type is LARGE and the letters well spaced, making the puzzles pleasing to work and easy on the eyes.

Enjoy another Inspirational Day!

HINTS TO SOLVE CRYPTOGRAMS

Cryptograms are fun to do and a great exercise for the mind. They are simply sentences in code.

One letter is replaced by another, throughout that particular puzzle. No letter will represent itself.

For example:

T H A T

P S M P

Here the P stands for T, the S stands for H and so on...The code remains the same throughout each particular puzzle.

Whereas, in another puzzle:

T H A T

V L C V

The V stands for T, the L stands for H ....

The frequency of letters occurring in the English language is as follows: E T A O N S and I.

Located at the top of each page is:

A B C D E F G H I J K L M N O P Q R S T U V W X Y Z

This can be used to count or eliminate letters used, as well as identifying the most common and frequently used letters.

A single letter word will be either an A or an I.

In a two letter words, one letter must be a vowel: as, to, an, do, we, or, it, is and so on....

Common three letter words: the, and, any, are, was, you, one, not, why…

Solving cryptograms relies on trial and error. So sharpen your pencil and have a good eraser on hand.

You have the clues in the back of the book to help get you started.

When all else fails, if you are *really* stuck, the answers are back there too.

ABCDEFGHIJKLMNOPQRSTUVWXYZ

1) S UXSP JO KXW SPDSCO
HQSKW WX IQ YQSRZQE, JW
XLWQK OQYTQO OJHNPC SO
OXHQWZJKU WX SJH SW.

IYVRQ PQQ

---

2) IQKBFNK. XKF RD. BOE
QKJGOE VDCQZKXW FNBF
FNGZ LKQV JDJKOF GZ FNK
DOXV DOK VDC UODP VDC
NBLK WDQ ZCQK.

DYQBN PGOWQKV

---

3) NBB ZRJV BG Y UBBE
NVLIU JYI HD FBIEDSGRO.

ZYD FDMN

ABCDEFGHIJKLMNOPQRSTUVWXYZ

4) AWYROZS YE EYGIRD KUS

MIIMZKOVYKD KM TSLYV

WLWYV, KUYE KYGS GMZS

YVKSRRYLSVKRD. USVZD AMZX

---

5) NR'B HODHVB RLU ONRROU

PUYNBNFXB RLHR LHEU RLU

ZNKKUBR NQAHYR.

QHMW YJZHX

---

6) MEG NYCL JOL NS SAYVAYR

MEG CAKAMF NS MEG

DNFFATCG AF TL RNAYR

TGLNYV MEGK AYMN MEG

AKDNFFATCG.

OZMEWZ U. UCOZPG

A B C D E F G H I J K L M N O P Q R S T U V W X Y Z

7) KH CDS YDV'E EAKVW

OPOUC YFC KX F TDDY YFC,

LSXE EUC BKXXKVT DVO.

JFPOEE UDQOUE

8) RFH'W IAKITW HFW WF EI

GLSGDR. SIGC TFMSGXI DP

EIDHX PTGSIR WF RIGWY

GHR XFDHX GYIGR GHJOGJ.

ESIWW ODCPFH

9) EVNZDEI LBDSCP PXSG-

XPNXXH OEC PXSG-

WVEGDCXEWX SDUX

OWWVHKSDPZHXEN.

NZVHOP WOQSJSX

3

ABCDEFGHIJKLMNOPQRSTUVWXYZ

10) TKWAER TALNKWXL
LATHGC TXKEL CFO KZX
GXKZEAER BKLNXZ.

QXLNFE D. KRFZ

11) HJMFBLSC NU J
LCJDRMNHNYSC XNLB DT
UNES SIISPLU.

JCDTHE B. FHJUFTX

12) CDE LU AJE XD HJAEDAE
EJ SFVE FAO UDD SRFE SVCC
RFQQDA, XLE BVKD LU ERD
ODEDZYVAFEVJA EJ YFTD
ERD ZVBRE ERVABU RFQQDA.

RJZFHD YFAA

13) PZ OSB KWLY YS VWUX

OSBJ GJXWVC HSVX YJBX, YQX

ZPJCY YQPLE OSB QWTX YS

GS PC KWUX BA.   N.V. ASKXJ

---

14) BQLHD FQL HMX OB UMY'B

WD ALYD MKD ZHZMPPX

OYBDKKZVBDA WX LBQDKH

ALOYR OB. IMEDH M. WMPAFOY

---

15) QI JND ZVQBATVJ FN SAPB

JND FN PLF JND'WT UNNF PB

SAPB JND FN, PLF BWJ BN ZT

P FTMTLB KTWGNL, JND MPL

GDMMTTF.

     OQMAPTV KPBWQMC RPLL

ABCDEFGHIJKLMNOPQRSTUVWXYZ

16) XZV XZOFL RPD ZSCV XP
TV EQVESQVI KPQ OH XZSX
PXZVQ EVPEWV IPF'X SWASRH
IQVSY RPDQ IQVSY.

WOFIS QPFHXSIX

---

17) E XRFJT FX E ABQDT IMEI
XTIX TDTQSIMFZH XIQEFHMI.

GMSJJFX UFJJTQ

---

18) FHMG ZU RGW ERTWEE
RGYR IWZIDW UWWD KZWEC'R
MZFW UTZF GYQOCX RZZ
FHMG RZ KZ. OR MZFWE UTZF
CZR UOCOEGOCX BGYR RGWS
ERYTRWK.   KYQOK YDDWC

ABCDEFGHIJKLMNOPQRSTUVWXYZ

19) MAIAK LAFF GARGFA SRT LR OR LSPMQH. LAFF LSAD TSYL LR OR YMO LSAZ TPFF HJKGKPHA ZRJ TPLS LSAPK PMQAMJPLZ.

QARKQA H. GYLLRM

20) WSMBERS SEGBM, PBE UZD OBYWVD OBGV BY WSV XBMOW KIBXO WSZW ITYV CVITHVMO. ZDC BDUV PBE YTDC IZERSWVM, DB GZWWVM SBX FZTDYEI PBEM OTWEZWTBD GTRSW KV, PBE UZD OEMHTHV TW.

KTII UBOKP

A B C D E F G H I J K L M N O P Q R S T U V W X Y Z

21) RSX JSF'W FZZJ HFRUSJR

WS WZGG RSX VPS RSX HKZ

SK VPHW RSX HKZ. RSX HKZ

VPHW RSX HKZ!

DSPF GZFFSF

---

22) EXMFQEB KMXWK MFH OPE

CFX IHKQAHK MX PLFQHZH.

HZHAT XVKMPLUH QK KQOWUT

P LXRAKH MX IHZHUXW FQK

PLFQHZHOHEM ORKLUH.

QM'K P KMAHEBMFHEQEB

XD FQK WXCHAK XD

PLLXOWUQKFOHEM.

HAQL VRMMHACXAMF

ABCDEFGHIJKLMNOPQRSTUVWXYZ

23) FU MID IYQM AI OZJR MID

EYIO MID SJY AI- MID YKTKH

AI TKHM XDSZ.   RIX EHJDGK

---

24) SXQM CSJ OMLGHQM

XMTHREIM RZSJTZRD UERZ

LSDEREIM SXMD, CSJ'GG

DRHOR ZHIEXT LSDEREIM

OMDJGRD.   UEGGEM XMGDSX

---

25) SRZ RNTTUGZJJ KI DKCM

YUIZ FZTZGFJ CTKG SRZ

HCNYUSD KI DKCM SRKCBRSJ;

SRZMZIKMZ BCNMF

NQQKMFUGBYD.

ANMQCJ NCMZYUCJ

ABCDEFGHIJKLMNOPQRSTUVWXYZ

26) U ATLMS HC AWHKUKTDTZN
TR QHWZS U AHJLE HC
AXWSUAR.   PUBXR ZSJWKXW

27) MLMAN QMAIPD, ZYY RCM
MLMDRI PB NPJA YHBM ZAM
RCMAM EMKZJIM NPJ CZLM
SAZUD RCMX RCMAM. UCZR
NPJ KCPPIM RP SP UHRC
RCMX HI JQ RP NPJ.

                    AHKCZAS EZKC

28) OQW DTJR HQ GZFN EQZIE
HQQ BTG HQ MZFUQJRG AWFH
DQY BTG OQW UTI GRTXXO
EQ.   MGTNR

A B C D E F G H I J K L M N O P Q R S T U V W X Y Z

29) BGY XPN BZ QYB JBPIBYT

FJ BZ LRFB BPUCFWQ PWT

VYQFW TZFWQ. XPUB TFJWYN

---

30) WGNQQ MFFMW MERF NHF

SFOOFH OANR LHFNO MFFMW

IQNRRFM. IFOFH GNHWANQQ

---

31) XASVB BEDB, MRX CNSXC

FEA BEIIAO EO JRPX CRPF.

IXASY IAAZ, MRX ALAXJ

IXASY ZXAVAIAC NBA DRSF.

            ZSYAFS LSPFF CNSXX

---

32) IRA WCH CJTCIP EZWRBZ

EZKKZU.   KXFZU TRRVP

ABCDEFGHIJKLMNOPQRSTUVWXYZ

33) QAV LAI'E LFNFYAJ
HAVCXZF PQ PFUIZ DXJJQ
UI QAVC CFYXEUAIMDUJM
FNFCQLXQ. QAV LFNFYAJ UE
PQ MVCNUNUIZ LURRUHVYE
EUOFM XIL HDXYYFIZUIZ
XLNFCMUEQ.   FJUHVCVM

---

34) PAE QAT'Z TFFQ IGZFY ZA
KFFR ROUF PAE'YF QYAITOTD,
QA PAE?   BAQO LOSAERZ

---

35) EWXG EX SYC P OMBMC
ZG EWPC EX EMOO IZ, EX
SYC P OMBMC ZG EWPC EX
NPG IZ.   NWPHOXD DNWEPF

ABCDEFGHIJKLMNOPQRSTUVWXYZ

36) JWD FADMJDHJ JWQDU

JWQH YBAOX WMH DNDA

SABXVZDX QH

SABZAMHJQCMJQBC, MCX

WD QH HJQOO MJ OMAFD.

      WDCAT YWDDOJDA HWMY

---

37) RE RDYMN REE WEMX

PUEVR AEYMX P RDYMX

EORJM UJKESJG YRG

VMAEYMX.   JBP IEVMX

---

38) BEC BH ADC OMCXACLA

RXVBM-LXYPEO PEYCEAPBEL

BH ABKXN PL ABTBMMBZ.

      YPEGCEA A. HBLL

ABCDEFGHIJKLMNOPQRSTUVWXYZ

39) WH ONNHKYEVDU ZIXOW
WUVQZD, BX KJDW QHW HQEF
ONW, PJW OEDH SIXOK; QHW
HQEF YEOQ, PJW OEDH
PXEVXGX.   OQOWHEX MIOQNX

---

40) VRN ZTZIMNPFVY NPCN FD
JCKZX KCV OZ KPCVYZX, OHN
VRNPFVY KCV OZ KPCVYZX
HVNFA FN FD JCKZX.

BCWZD C. OCAXUFV

---

41) KCM CEE MINJ LJINOEZT
ECTL CT EIHR CT MINJ HZU
MZCJ'T JZTIENLQIHT.

PIZM CYCKT

ABCDEFGHIJKLMNOPQRSTUVWXYZ

42) CVFPGBPFAZFR BGXAGBY EVF XJF SGPLY GB XJF RGGV XG NAYRGD.   DFVVK WVGNBF

43) RS CQLCTR HGYC RS RFCIR XSM JSSN GA YSSHGAO IA OSLGVJ I ZMHH PSV'R OGR XSM ZCTIMAC XSM IFC I ECJCRIFGIV.   FSAIVVC ZIFF

44) QBDQCW IPZQOP BHVP Q ANJV- VPPL JQBF QUA NUTNGGBPA SU XZP WNTGQJP, INX LQAABP BHVP XZP APOHB NUAPTUPQXZ.

YQJSI F. ITQNAP

ABCDEFGHIJKLMNOPQRSTUVWXYZ

45) DMJJNDD XD G DLGLN FU
RXPK. XU AFM VGPL DMJJNDD,
DLGYL LBXPZXPI FU
AFMYDNQU GD G DMJJNDD.

         KY. HFAJN SYFLBNYD

---

46) VBGZ B EQBUEZ! BJJ
JNLZ NF B EQBUEZ. VQZ KBU
SQT XTZF VQZ LIOVQZFV NF
XZUZOBJJP VQZ TUZ SQT NF
SNJJNUX VT CT BUC CBOZ.

         CBJZ EBOUZXNZ

---

47) DMC TNI ZKTQ DMC
RIGOIAI DMCNBIGY QM RI.

         FTCGM JMIGKM

ABCDEFGHIJKLMNOPQRSTUVWXYZ

48) EYXT UWI UZAI GFVAI XB
URLI; CYFUMW, CIROI, FYS
IYPXH IGIZH LXLIYU XB RU.
YX RSVIYICC, YX SIVFH, YX
NZXMZFCURYFURXY; YIGIZ
NAU XBB URVV UXLXZZXT
TWFU HXA MFY SX UXSFH.

VXZS MWICUIZBRIVS

49) WD BKKX ODRE QMEEVMJK
YEVQQVAJ, TVWG HDUK VA
WGK TKNNVAJ LRX, TGKAKUKE
ODR'EK TEDAJ, MNQVW VW;
TGKAKUKE ODR'EK EVJGW,
IGRW RX.   DJNKA AMIG

ABCDEFGHIJKLMNOPQRSTUVWXYZ

50) XD TZJ GHUVR TZJF KXDU

IZVIUVRFPRXVW ZV LMPR

UYUFTZVU UKGU RMZJWMR

ZD TZJ, LZJKB TZJ DZFWUR

LMZ TZJ FUPKKT LUFU?

EZBX HXIZJKR

---

51) XAVN NXH UBA ZHEQJ

NXHP VYTJ. NXH OBLJ KX

VYLJ HR KX NXHP XIA

JGRJUKBKYXAC.

IXVTQBAQ RHUD

---

52) VDQ JDRP YD R

LCGAWDVCP RAN ACQ R

MRXVDP. RAQUCAZ PCYYXAW

ABCDEFGHIJKLMNOPQRSTUVWXYZ

53) OD ZFIW ZQTOFIWT QT

PSZFA; OD TOSZGBW QT

XDZZDAUBFXW; OD GW FGBW

OD BFSHP FO MDSKTWBJ QT

ZFOSKQOM. CQBBQFZ F. CFKR

54) MLWOGYLX ZDOM GDL

JDCO TWDC FXSMKJUQ

JUFUJKLS. KL JDCOM TWDC

UG KGZDCKLUHQO VKQQ.

CUXULCU YUGZXK

55) CDNCPD PNYD NUBDEO

FNU RNE IBN UBDH SED KWU

RNE BNI UBDH VSTD UBDV

RDDP. LEILF RDJDEVSF

A B C D E F G H I J K L M N O P Q R S T U V W X Y Z

56) H IUQQIR IUR UF IUTR

H IUQQIR DLROKHKBG UQ

WARFK'Q QHTR IAKO VRSALR

RERLGAKR TKAYF.

B. F. IRYUF

---

57) PODDXPP LXVIP BVKRIW

JBX DTOSVWX, JBX

AXJXSLRIVJRTI, VIA JBX

ERQQ JT UXDTLX JBX HXSPTI

NTO UXQRXKX NTO EXSX

LXVIJ JT UX.

WXTSWX PBXXBVI

---

58) ZWQ OAHBZ RPZT YO VYXQ

AB ZY VABZQI. FDPV ZAVVASW

ABCDEFGHIJKLMNOPQRSTUVWXYZ

59) HPQV AGL'WQ CQQV

XQAGVZ AGLTCQDR, BPQV AGL

KIA RYVZ, JQIOQ GR KYVZ YC

HIYBYVU BPQTQ.

UQGTUQ PITTYCGV

---

60) GYGQMVNJOR MCB UC

IQGIEQGF MCB XCQ VNG

OGAV VNJOR.   WCNO EPGZ

---

61) DJZQ Z YFQG JIWZP

THFPLM XZP'Q HOXJZPLH

YSETKHWM. HUHSGEPH CPEDM

HOZXQKG JED QE MEKUH QJH

EQJHS RHKKED'M.

EKFP WFKKHS

ABCDEFGHIJKLMNOPQRSTUVWXYZ

62) M'WZ KZZY OKPUTBAZTR
AZLLMNMZE ZWZLR IUIZYA UN
IR TMNZ - OYE M'WZ YZWZL
TZA MA CZZD IZ NLUI EUMYX
O PMYXTZ AVMYX M QOYAZE
AU EU.   XZULXMO U'CZZNNZ

---

63) SK RKQ ANQ JNYQNOSWJY
SHYWEEKHRQTNRQY
KBNOYCWSKZ KR QKTKOOKZY
SONWTY PNLWVYN JKVO
AHUN HY AHFN W THOOKO,
HU JKV FNNE YTHAHRD HQ
YTHANY OHDCQ PWLF WQ
JKV...YK, FNNE YTHAHRD.

                    VRFRKZR

ABCDEFGHIJKLMNOPQRSTUVWXYZ

64) JKASA UQ ZW AEUBAZXA JKFJ JKA JWZNOA UQ XWZZAXJAB JW JKA DSFUZ.

ISFZT JHNAS

---

65) VBNNMVV TV GF ZM XMCVBOMH EFG VF XBNR ZQ GRM WFVTGTFE GRCG FEM RCV OMCNRMH TE ITPM CV ZQ GRM FZVGCNIMV SRTNR RM RCV FLMONFXM.

ZFFAMO G. SCVRTEKGFE

---

66) YJQ FRDDQPY VRPE KTA BHM YHEQ RP YT YHEQ MT VRPE.   CHVE WABEQVFQVD

23

ABCDEFGHIJKLMNOPQRSTUVWXYZ

67) XYH XYGHH RGHQX

HZZHJXAQUZ XP QWYAHKH

QJLXYAJR EPGXY EYAUH QGH,

OAGZX, YQGM EPGN; ZHWPJM,

ZXAWN-XP-AXAKHJHZZ;

XYAGM, WPBBPJ ZHJZH.

XYPBQZ HMAZPJ

68) XAK PWQGR FKG F RAO

EXEFP XS EZG IZXWIGR MG

ZFQG OFYG.

YK. MFLTG M. YLGK

69) UMJEPUN EIX CMSQ

XJSQUNJE JEIU RPSQ

UQHQXXPJV.   QZPHJQJBX

ABCDEFGHIJKLMNOPQRSTUVWXYZ

70) RQWDZEZF OPLFXZ JPL
BZOHBZ LVPY, DQZFZ HX
WIRWJX XPCZPYZ DP DZII JPL
DQWD JPL WFZ RFPYN. DQZFZ
WFZ WIRWJX BHMMHOLIDHZX
WFHXHYN, RQHOQ DZCVD JPL
DP SZIHZEZ DQWD JPLF
OFHDHOX WFZ FHNQD. DP CWV
PLD W OPLFXZ PM WODHPY
WYB MPIIPR HD DP WY ZYB
FZGLHFZX OPLFWNZ.

FWIVQ RWIBP ZCZFXPY

71) CI UKZVNK VZ CI IOCBVR;
CI BZDVNK VZ CI BXTVKLK.

PBJKZ BWWKR

A B C D E F G H I J K L M N O P Q R S T U V W X Y Z

72) LBGLKKLPGL UI PXQ Y
IUPDMKYZ YGQ, EMQ Y
TYEUQ. SXM YZL VTYQ SXM
ZLNLYQLHKS HX.

ITYWMUKKL X'PLYK

73) GCFQH QCAVFQH FR TBMS
VYMG AC GC...SCK QBTBM
PQCJ JVBQ SCK'MB UFQFRVBG.

XBRXFB QFBXRBQ

74) OHBKYSXY KP PANYBJKSF
VAD HUNKTY KS BJY UTKQYT
CYJKSU VAD, HSU PXATS KS
BJY ASY HJYHU.

NHX NXXEYHTV

ABCDEFGHIJKLMNOPQRSTUVWXYZ

75) B KPEJTPEQLO QL FSO BTF
PI VQYQVQCZ B KBWO QC
LXKS B MBR FSBF OYOTRPCO
HOGQOYOL SO SBL FSO
HQZZOLF JQOKO.

GXVMQZ OTSBTV

---

76) WR WZ BKR JMATGZM
RVWBCZ TDM OWQQWAGFR
RVTR NM OK BKR OTDM, WR
WZ JMATGZM NM OK BKR OTDM
RVTR RVMS TDM OWQQWAGFR.

ZMBMAT

---

77) JSRRWJJ FJ IWQWEIWEG
LE WOOLTG.   JLQXLRKWJ

27

ABCDEFGHIJKLMNOPQRSTUVWXYZ

78) KOY LUS DYRGYK UZ

TUVY UD KOMK KOYGY UD

ZP LUS DYRGYK. HOMKYIYG

WPNG SPMT, WPN RMZ SYK

KOYGY UV WPN'GY HUTTUZS

KP HPGX.   PQGMO HUZVGYW

---

79) TESTUVTGQT VL CRT

IGJP LQRIIJ KUIA XRVQR

GI IGT TWTU MUDNFDCTL.

                    TWDG TLDU

---

80) BPA LGQB VKWWAR-

DFGT FHAHAODNQNBA GE K

EHNATR NQ KT KVVAQQNIWA

AKH.   LKZK KTJAWGD

ABCDEFGHIJKLMNOPQRSTUVWXYZ

81) RBB WPEXBTFG XTAEFT
GFRBBTP DH LEI QEK'J QEQYT
JUTF XIJ AEKHPEKJ JUTF.

ZDBBDRF H. URBGTL

---

82) QX QW QBENJXGKX XTGX
INZ JLVNUKQSL INZJ
EJNUJLWW GKM XGFL EJQML
QK INZJ GVVNBECQWTBLKXW.
WTGJL INZJ GVTQLRLBLKXW
PQXT NXTLJW. OJGU G
CQXXCL. XTL JLVNUKQXQNK
GKM WZEENJX ND XTNWL
GJNZKM INZ QW KZJXZJQKU.

JNWLBGJQL JNWWLXXQ

ABCDEFGHIJKLMNOPQRSTUVWXYZ

83) YGZ GZZAX XYRZVLDGW
VY EZQDZBZ DG, XYRZVLDGW
CYF JLDKL YGZ KPG LPBZ
JLYQZ-LZPFVZA ZGVLIXDPXR.
YGZ GZZAX VY CZZQ VLPV
YGZ'X QDCZ LPX RZPGDGW,
VLPV YGZ DX GZZAZA DG
VLDX JYFQA. LPGGPL XZGZXL

---

84) TGLS YTV ELVECL ULIJUL
YV HLY X UJZVPIL, JY JAS'Y
X AJHS YGXY YGLB "UVS'Y
QSULPAYXSU" VSL XSVYGLP,
OQY X AJHS YGXY YGLB
GXZL, XY CXAY, OLHQS YV.
                    GLCLS PVTCXSU

ABCDEFGHIJKLMNOPQRSTUVWXYZ

85) HI PMVFV XFV PMHOSW

DBA QBO'P KHZV HO PMV

YBFKQ DBA SFVY AE HO, NXZV

DBAF BYO KHIV QHIIVFVOP.

QXLV PMBNXW

86) JOFMQ IB JDWIOQ.

BVVBMITQDIR PBTJY LO

AQBPADQH FI RBTM YBBM

COMR WBEIJR.   EMFQA IRHOM

87) EOA SQA OUZG LUI

WODFOHFCY FC ISQV LVOUKE.

PCSJ JFAGSQA U LSQWA AGUA

ISQ JOVO KULO XSV UKUBFCY

AGFCYE.   TSEG GFCLE

A B C D E F G H I J K L M N O P Q R S T U V W X Y Z

88) ONZ KZPD FQD RXUNCUQH

DN GVUQ VX RKTVBD. XN NXQ

RP RKTSQPPQH ARDG DGQ

ANX – CNPD SQBNSH NL DGQ

SQLQSQQ.   MNGX G. GNCBNKY

---

89) WO MGSUYKQI QLKPED KP

NKMI CUP'Q AUDQ GPO WUPIO.

KQ'D YIGNNO ANIGY QLGQ QLI

WUDQ FYIAKUVD YIDUVYAI BI

GNN LGSI KD QKWI.

DQISI TUXD

---

90) LUW PCYY AJEJF PCA CN

LUW AJEJF GJRCA.

XJYJA FUPYHAV

ABCDEFGHIJKLMNOPQRSTUVWXYZ

91) VHCW HQ VHIW J SWL-
QMWWX UHKPKVW. GRQS RC
ZQ DJNW BWJYQ EW LWNWY
ZQW.   KDJYVWQ G. QKDZVF

92) ZUR NJXA OGQMG XUK
HZ YGQYYQXVJXV KWG
MJYMRIDKQXMGD UN ZURY
CJNG, HRK HZ YGQCJFJXV
SWU ZUR QYG QK KWG
AGGOGDK CGBGC.

                GMPWQYK KUCCG

93) NBFBE RTMN JUAQZPA
CTPHQABX YTDB ZEB JBTD.

                LZBC HZZRYTE

ABCDEFGHIJKLMNOPQRSTUVWXYZ

94) TRXNULB UL Q KIRRA
NQRXIQXT. SBQS TYJNQURL
DBA DT JQFW VIF EQF VR SBT
CFUZTDQA QRC CFUZT VIF
EQF VR SBT JQFWDQA.

GQFW XFQLLV

95) VS MSKSW GMCV ADS
VCWAD CP VZASW AQXX ADS
VSXX QF OWT.

ADCJZF PEXXSW

96) IXQ KWV OVAVW YXX XJT
YX UVY KOXYSVW PXKJ XW
YX TWVKG K OVN TWVKG.

JVU ZWXNO

ABCDEFGHIJKLMNOPQRSTUVWXYZ

97) CD'M DAH LPBMDZBD
ZBR RHDHIQCBHR HEEPID
DAZD SIHZTM RPFB ZUU
IHMCMDZBLH, MFHHWM
ZFZG ZUU PSMDZLUHM.

LUZORH Q. SICMDPU

98) BUU KQBHMJC BIJ LNIJ
NI UJCC YDHMJX GDYQ
LJUBHKQNUZ, WNI GQBY GJ
BIJ UJBFDHM EJQDHX DC VBIY
NW NRICJUFJC.   BLJUDB EBII

99) WOUI OM YVI MGC DU
HWW FDGQ XVDOXIM.

HWJIQY XHCGM

ABCDEFGHIJKLMNOPQRSTUVWXYZ

100) JKQ HYDJ VXIYPJVXRJQ
JKBXO JKRJ KRNNQXD JY R
NQPDYX ZKY IQRPD IRBFVPQ
BD JKRJ KQ FBHBJD KBHDQFI
CM CQEYHBXO RIPRBS JY
JPM RXMJKBXO XQZ.

FQY CVDEROFBR

---

101) BAKU SHF JYIXY YH
OKQKZHV SHFX VHBKXJ HE
KTVIYAS IUO GTILGUIYGHU,
YAK BAHZK BHXZO HVKUJ FV
YH SHF.   JFJIU JIXIUOHU

---

102) F MTA XRFUSO GX F
MTA OTVPBSO.   J. X. BSIGX

ABCDEFGHIJKLMNOPQRSTUVWXYZ

103) XIDKU FRMC SREUF IEQ
FRM'CU REHF RMK RJ SREUF,
ZMK XIDKU FRMC KWSU IEQ
FRM'TU HRDK I LICK RJ FRMC
HWJU.   SWGAIUH HUZRUMJ

104) CIA'W WJN WI PMOKJF
IKW QLYW IWLFJ XFIXTF
QYAW WI LFYJ PJIU NIK;
PMOKJF IKW QLYW NIK LYSF
WI BYN.

          GYJGYJY ZMAOBITSFJ

105) KNEE KZN KFPKZ, MF
HMBNMRN LQEE KNEE QK CMF
WMP.   HKNIZTRQN YENQR

37

ABCDEFGHIJKLMNOPQRSTUVWXYZ

106) PY DUZTC PY PITCF
GTPI KHJKYLU TL PY UCPUJ
PIU JSCFL YM PIYLU LPJYCZ
YCUL GIY YCWV JURYZCTAU
MSTWHJU SL YCU YM PIU
KSPIGSVL PY SPPSTCBUCP.

QSBUL SWWUC

---

107) MCF LFKW UCOS
MCFDKSUR NSRCDS MCF
UCOS VQCWBSD. NM
VAASZWPQI MCFDKSUR VQX
RFUUM NSPQI YBVW MCF VDS,
MCFD KPLZUS ZDSKSQAS
AVQ LVES CWBSDK BVZZM.

LPIQCQ LAUVFIBUPQ

ABCDEFGHIJKLMNOPQRSTUVWXYZ

108) LK PGFWC'Z HYZU TR
WSS PULKJ PGG NYEU, ZRRJ
PGG NYEU, TWKP PGG NYEU
WKF QGHMRP WXGYP PUR
OGC GQ OYZP XRLKM.

REJUWHP PGSSR

---

109) TNISV VFD RQHGDS JA
VFD XUNCDHB, SDEDH JA VFD
UDQEDB VFQV XQUU. TNISV
ANIH UKXD CKVF BZKUDB QSG
SNV VFD VDQHB VFQV HNUU.

ISYSNCS

---

110) VFL BOVOJL KT YA
DSSDJVOAKVW.   M. B. RYJL

ABCDEFGHIJKLMNOPQRSTUVWXYZ

111) ZSW XOCWXZ PEN ZG
WXYEIW ERFLWZN ERM
MWQWEZ MWXIELC LX EYZLGR.
MG, MGR'Z MPWAA.

JLYSEWA HGXWISXGR

---

112) PMZNG AU VINGAVC, XJN
NI RAHM PMWMZNMP ZVP
AVCRIQAIJU AU NI PAM PZARK.

VZDIRMIV XIVZDZQNM

---

113) KML WELDKLXK INXKDOL
TPS GDQ IDOL NQ BNCL NX
KP GPQKNQSDBBT FL DCEDNV
TPS ANBB IDOL PQL.

LBFLEK MSFFDEV

ABCDEFGHIJKLMNOPQRSTUVWXYZ

114) ZOB TNMZ JTSNYZKHZ
MZNYL XB'AA BWBY XYJZB JH
AJPB JM NGY NXH-HNZ XJZO
JHU, VGZ XJZO NGY EKJAL
RONJRBM.

YJROKYE SKGA BWKHM

---

115) H TVBIIU OAF'Q QDHFS
IHYV HW BRAPQ QDV H-MAPIO-
DBJV-RVVFW. IHYV HW AFIU
BRAPQ QDV H-QTHVO-QA-OA.
H OAF'Q KHFO QDV YBHIPTV
RPQ H MBF'Q HKBLHFV QDBQ
H'O YATLHJV KUWVIY HY H
OHOF'Q QTU.

FHSSH LHAJBFFH

ABCDEFGHIJKLMNOPQRSTUVWXYZ

116) PIRME SYGEXC, SZ
DPMEXGEX WPY GEEYB
MWWGWIHYC KL WPYGB
RGEHC, DME DPMEXY WPY
KIWYB MCQYDWC KL WPYGB
FGTYC.   VGFFGMR AMRYC

---

117) RL EROM JZUE URP IMD
NXZD URP NZLD, ZLJ RL
RDXMGE, URP IMD NXZD URP
LMMJ. XPLDMG E. DXROYERL

---

118) JNCSC'H PM ZMMD
DFBC WP MDG ZMMD - RMK
TWP'J ECWJ COQCSFCPTC.
                UWTME A. ESWKGC

ABCDEFGHIJKLMNOPQRSTUVWXYZ

119) MIU KUEM ZDR MB
SBJPCJSU D OBBG MIDM IU CE
ZXBJA CE MB GUM ICQ IDPU
ICE BZJ ZDR.   NBEI KCGGCJAE

---

120) LOQ PNEENAJAQGG LY
BVVQDL ZQGDYAGNCNENLI
WYZ YAQ'G YPA ENWQ NG
LOQ GYRZVQ WZYX PONVO
GQEW-ZQGDQVL GDZNAJG.

HYBA MNMNYA

---

121) IBWKZHBS WRQ NLIDDW
XIBK, WRQ GIB IKKIHB, HY
WRQ NLIDDW SR IYKLN HK.

CN. XIWBL X. CWLN

ABCDEFGHIJKLMNOPQRSTUVWXYZ

122) LEQ HSQKH UW HUFDO
K LKIB JIQI JM NUSQ LFNQ
KDH QDQSOG LEKD HUFDO
LEQ LKIB FLIQZW.

SFLK QNNQLL

123) THOORVN ORCRV SWHP,
EOQ SWHPPRVN ORCRV THO.

CHOGR DABZEVQH

124) RK FRU ILCUYN
XHIHDKQZIW QKKX QKTKY
XKNGLHY; EUY LII ZRHQDN
LYK LSSUJGIHNRKX CW
XHIHDKQSK LQX ILCUY.

JKQLQXKY

ABCDEFGHIJKLMNOPQRSTUVWXYZ

125) NHENWH BKGQ ZEYWP
PMSSHHR DHSYMPH GQHO
XIEB BQHLH GQHO'LH ZEKIZ.

HYLW IKZQGKIZYWH

---

126) IXS ALY QFRUQB
AXTKGLFY XB GXXH MXB
XKKXBRSYFRI FY QCQBI
KBXWGQT. F KBQMQB
XKKXBRSYFRI.

KLSG XBMLGQL

---

127) QMDK NMJNTJMQKE
CXBDB. QRMQ XB ATXQK
EXVVKCKOQ VCYF SKXOL
CMBR. LKYCLK B. GMQQYO

128) FR VCR FPVU FR

WCRURTY UL KR, BL FR

JABU KR IVCRMAZ VKLAU

FPVU FR WCRURTY UL KR.

HACU ELTTRXAU

---

129) JXB EBWA PLFWA KC

QVX JXB FCYTTJ YFC, AVCG

NX QVYA JXB GCCN AX NX,

LG XFNCF AX VYOC QVYA

JXB QYGA. EYFUYFCA JXBGU

---

130) IMACVIH HQYUA XUZ

YNYQ UKCVYNYR XVACMBA

YIACBZVUZD.

XVPPVUD XQVHPYT OQ.

ABCDEFGHIJKLMNOPQRSTUVWXYZ

131) XUE TUY'Z SKOM ZU BMM
ZSM JSUQM BZKPDAKBM, FEBZ
ZKWM ZSM IPDBZ BZMC.

HKDZPY QEZSMD WPYL, FD.

---

132) JTQ OPJ RC BCACDKCB
DG JTQ LNQWL LTT OQAV, RQL
JTQ YDSS SDKC DI LTNOCIL
DG JTQ BT ITL LNQWL CITQXV.

GNPIF ANPIC

---

133) PDCEP MGFJ VMINVNGP.
FOKN ZSQQNGE SP PZN FNINF
MK NINGPE, GMP MK HMDXE.
PDCEP VMINVNGP.

SFKDNX SXFND

ABCDEFGHIJKLMNOPQRSTUVWXYZ

134) SY ZFG WFGCX ZFG APK
PAAFDHRSEJ EFDBXJSKT,
XJBK ZFG APK'X PAAFDHRSEJ
SX. ZFG JPQB XF JPQB
AFKYSWBKAB SK ZFGM
PCSRSXZ, PKW XJBK CB XFGTJ
BKFGTJ XF YFRRFI XJMFGTJ.

                    MFEPRZK APMXBM

---

135) EKWXPSPF ALO'FP ZLDCZ
XKFLOZK DC ALOF IDUP,
JLC'X PSPF ZDSP OR.

                    NWFDWK BWFPA

---

136) D LXKARY BDY'O BPDYNX
DCC DO RYBX. AOXLPXY EHYN

ABCDEFGHIJKLMNOPQRSTUVWXYZ

137) NWLC ZVB WL

DJDGBPEWLX BVA HEVVTD

PV CV. DJDGB ZVQ,

GDMSPWVLTEWR, EVFD...WP'T

BVAG GDTRVLTWQWMWPB PV

MVJD WP, VG HESLXD WP.

HEAHU RSMSELWAU

138) KTT BKGGQKJOR KGO

VKWWN. QY'R TQXQPJ

YAJOYVOG KEYOGSKGCR YVKY

QR CQEEQUITY.   IPLPASP

139) VOO UOXTF JXBYZ GTXB

CVTWPU NX KYUWP.

YEUYPY G. DVTY

ABCDEFGHIJKLMNOPQRSTUVWXYZ

140) EG QIZK SV'F TAQM
ALKEIU AQ YV RHMMK SV
XQWZF RHCV H MLVAAK UQQF
AEDV.   VFEAR SRHLAQI

---

141) TMM JVCRYA VTKKBR
LDE T EBTADR, BUBR JVDWYV
CJ'A TR BJBERCJQ ADZBJCZBA
HBLDEB IB MBTER JVDAB
EBTADRA.   WRXRDIR

---

142) NETR XRTRO YVANZ.
DMVOVDGRO XRTRO SKAGZ.
VXH JAGM QVGARXDR VXH
QROZAZGRXDR, HORVPZ HE
DEPR GOKR. QRGR PVOVTADM

ABCDEFGHIJKLMNOPQRSTUVWXYZ

143) W QHCHP LPHRBHL ROEJD
XJFFHXX. W NEPTHL MEP WD.

HXDHH GRJLHP

144) OGQDI MJUMYJ EFUH
INJBD OIDJFKINO, LAI NQMMR
MJUMYJ QDJ INJ UFJO HNU
NQWJ QSSJMIJP INJBD VYQHO.

EBGU

145) CD XLJ'VV ALH FMHHVM
DLG KAXHICAS VMFF HIKA
XLJG RMFH, XLJ BCVV RM
KZKUMN KH BIKH XLJ QKA
KQQLZEVCFI CA XLJG VCPMF.

PCAQM VLZRKGNC

ABCDEFGHIJKLMNOPQRSTUVWXYZ

146) GZDDXGG GXXBG YM

NX DMHHXDYXJ YM ODYCMH.

GZDDXGGIZE QXMQEX SXXQ

BMPCHA. YVXR BOSX

BCGYOSXG, NZY YVXR

HXPXL TZCY.

W. KCEEOLJ BOLLCMYY

---

147) KAUHIXTPUM UT WUFH

ZLIHE, HCTUHA ZCXH JPCI

FHMJ.   TCZRHW GRJWHA

---

148) ADXORAM RF TDJW

ZWFHRECYNW XOCA

JWFHWEX YCFWZ DA QWCJ.

CNYWJX ECTPF

ABCDEFGHIJKLMNOPQRSTUVWXYZ

149) UVDDZUU CU IRXZ

KZXITSZSP FJZS LRV TDJCZGZ

CP FCPJRVP YZUPXRLCSE

LRVX KXCSDCKHZU.

FTHPZX DXRSQCPZ

---

150) RGFGW JRPGWWSIP

CUYGURG EUJRO TVMP NUS

CMJE AUSBER'P KG EURG.

MYGBJM GMWVMWP

---

151) JTUEU SHLUV O JNLU NZ

JTU OPPONEV HP LOZ GTUZ

TU LKVJ JOMU JTU XKCC XQ

JTU JONC OZR POSU JTU

VNJKOJNHZ.   G. S. PNUCRV

ABCDEFGHIJKLMNOPQRSTUVWXYZ

152) R BRVVS VMFYWL PY
LWE R VMFYWL PL R KMFERPL
YME WT KPFKZHYERLKMY,
AZE FREBMF R VMFYWL
UPEB R KMFERPL YME WT
REEPEZNMY.   BZOB NWULY

---

153) EZF KPESMPH CHBWZEI
JC EZF ZSGPK GBKU PMF KJE
CMJG YHFPISMF EJ YHFPISMF
DSE CMJG ZJYF EJ ZJYF.

                    IPGSFH XJZKIJK

---

154) RZGQ ZJE'H I AIHHQL
KG AZRQJHKEQJ, SDH KG
AKAQEHJ.   LKJQ OQEEQXF

155) HLLRJVTXW HZZ VUR WIIY
HXY EHY HEIFV OIGRIXR. TV'O
H WDRHV VUTXW VI HOJTDR
VI. VUR UHDY JHDV TO
HLVFHZZK YITXW TV.

OHDHU YROORX

---

156) DLR LRBRC LDEOQRP
AYIE YIP FRRL ZDLR; DLR QIL
DLWM PRR AYIE CRGIOLP ED
FR ZDLR.   GICOR QHCOR

---

157) JFZ CXL HPVL PN UFL
KLHU UFEBQH EB RENL HPVL
PN UFL UFEBQH UFCU FTXU
TH UFL VPHU?   CVZ ICYEH

ABCDEFGHIJKLMNOPQRSTUVWXYZ

158) EZR VUDUW AMBX RVQBX
EZR NQZJ QWEBVH.

MXGUWQ UBVNQUBV

---

159) HNLQ EIXF HQNFB NJR
RIXVZB, NJR JQD DIFCRB
DYCC IWQJ ZI EIX.

FIVQFZ SYEIBNSY

---

160) Z QMZS JSKT DKO QKL
TZQ OHNB QKL BZC NWZSWMC
WKCZQ.   RZSMD VZTP

---

161) XRMKCGABG KECC BEZG
DMI HMKGQ, TIV JFOQOJVGQ
QGNHGJV.   TQIJG CGG

A B C D E F G H I J K L M N O P Q R S T U V W X Y Z

162) OGFI QHSF BIMTBA PME YMOI PME GXUF COM TGMHTFA - ACXP YMOI MZ VFC ED.

CMN BZXEAF

---

163) OJGIG DQ THRE THG XGIQTH BJT KTPRF GCGI UZYG ETP JZXXE, ZHF OJZO XGIQTH DQ ETP.

FZCDF WPIHQ

---

164) CNSH'U WJB VGJRB BTH KHJKCH ATJ VOB BJ PJRD SVOH. NB'U VGJRB BTH KHJKCH ATJ DHQVNW BDRH GHTNWZ PJRD GVOM.

VWJWPQJRU

ABCDEFGHIJKLMNOPQRSTUVWXYZ

165) EDC SXGY EDKE PBGNI
LXVM EMVC ZKWBPL BI GXE
XGC XZ SPXXY, SVE XZ
MCITCFE KGY AXL BG CKFD
XEDCM'I PBZC. MBFDKMY SKFD

166) GKKGFDSVLDLBM DG
WLVA ABBKBF KGQBFM QLDZLV
GSFMBECBM UGOB QZBV ELWB
MBBOM OGMD UZREEBVXLVX.

                    IGMBKZ UROKJBEE

167) JFH GDRJ VGQDNJOUJ
JFVUA VU WDGGTUVWOJVDU
VR FHONVUA IFOJ VRU'J
ROVB.   QHJHN BNTWEHN

A B C D E F G H I J K L M N O P Q R S T U V W X Y Z

168) ZHA CSHCWS OYSJO MHN
QF OZSQY GJYUJ. ZHA MHN
YSJXO QF MHNYF.

VY. AJMDS A. VMSY

---

169) MQ MK WPQ KP OAUZ PAJ
NJMBWG'K ZBSL QZDQ ZBSLK
AK DK QZB UPWNMGBWUB PN
QZBMJ ZBSL.   BLMUAJAK

---

170) JUVJNU VZPUC KTM PFTP
EVPOGTPOVC XVUKC'P NTKP.
IUNN, CUOPFUA XVUK
QTPFOCH - PFTP'K IFM IU
AUDVEEUCX OP XTONM.

YOH YOHNTA

ABCDEFGHIJKLMNOPQRSTUVWXYZ

171) DQXTM QE FWJ CQTOEJB,
EQF FWJ AJMFSEVFSQE. CQB
SM DQTEA EQF SE DSESMWSEY
VE VXFSISFB RTF SE AQSEY
SF.   YOJY VEAJOMQE

---

172) TXFPWVU FM BZC CZ YU
TUXVUE. FC FM TVZD TXFPWVU
CJXC DZMC RVZSCJ AZDUM.

                        EUU JZAN

---

173) AJXI FRI AJRA HKEX
UF NKPX UNBKPARWA AJRW
NKWXI, SCA JREX IKC XEXP
APUXY AK BRI IKCP SUHHF
TUAJ R JCL?   RWKWINKCF

60

ABCDEFGHIJKLMNOPQRSTUVWXYZ

174) DH UQS FDWV RQFA BXC
GDJOFDU QG WJGC UQS NSHB
HNCWW BXC OQHCH, GQO UQS
QAWU PCB BQ KWDU QAC
OQSAR.   LCA XQPDA

---

175) AH BGF SG IYTM BGF'NR
TJITBU SGER, BGF'JJ XRM
IYTM BGF'NR TJITBU XGMMRE.
                    TEMYGEB QGDDAEU

---

176) FUEC KBYC ZBTCJ
OENCFKG, MNFIBEF SLWWCUJ
BU QKLJINWR KNRIFJ. NQ GBE
ICLU SCKKJ, RCF GBEU CLUJ
ZICZXCH.   CUNZI JCRLK

177) UZVCHCMQ RDV UNBBAUU
XCZEDNZ EFVT XDVS CU KCSA
ZVJCMQ ZD EFVHAUZ XEAVA
JDN EFHAM'Z OKFMZAT.

TFHCT YKJ

---

178) KG UXMK YWKY UI
XMFMJRZMX KGX ZHY UGYR
KEYURG UI TRDM UTZRDYKGY
YWKG KG UXMK YWKY MSUIYI
RGJA KI KG UXMK.   OHXXWK

---

179) QB'T BLY TQANZY
BLQUET QU ZQPY BLXB XSY
BLY AJTB YIBSXJSWQUXSO.

NXDZJ GJYZLJ

ABCDEFGHIJKLMNOPQRSTUVWXYZ

180) ATMH TG ATWH Q PITO.
NIS PQO GLHOE TC QON XQN
NIS XTGV, KSC NIS IOAN
GLHOE TC IOPH.

ATAATQO ETPWGIO

---

181) QCA DGDWMAFKQO AFHA
EHQ TD ECJQADZ ECJQAR,
HQZ QCA DGDWMAFKQO AFHA
ECJQAR EHQ TD ECJQADZ.

HITDWA DKQRADKQ

---

182) DOYN TOJ ACPRCLC RO
SYBIECPZ, TOJ NUTG YGUCIE
GUROD NYO'G JREGBIA SYB.

NRPPRTV ZCTGUCI

ABCDEFGHIJKLMNOPQRSTUVWXYZ

183) HXYYSLR MV QLA

ELXAJ JFBMQI MH MA SLYV

QLA MQGZWSY AJY HXYYSLR

AL RFCY RMVAFCYV.

RFJFARF IFQSJM

---

184) JI NZWRAX MWY AIY

WRE TIHEN ZWAX RN DHPG

TEWB VRENRQMS WRE ZWVIN.

CWZM T. GIMMIXF

---

185) UF FCSJN CN RGXW

XAGTCVJ FA WCLJ FTUJM

CKM QCUOJM CN UF MAJN FA

WCLJ FTUJM CKM NGXXJJMJM.

CKKJ RATTAH OUKMZJTVW

ABCDEFGHIJKLMNOPQRSTUVWXYZ

186) FRVVRVZ RIV'G
LBLXUGJRVZ, DNG FMVGRVZ
GY FRV RI.   BRVQL WYCDMXSR

---

187) FNTXT SXT YG RSDK
FNBDLY FNSF QT QBYN QT
NSZ ZGDT KTYFTXZSK, YG
VTQ FNSF QT VTTI IBPT ZGBDL
FGZSK.   RBLDGD REISWLNIBD

---

188) ZMGJDFR DVS'F FYM
CGR RTE CDVY FYDSLV FT AM,
STZ FYM CGR FYMR GXXMGZ
FT AM, AEF FYM CGR FYMR
GQFEGJJR GZM.

ZTAMZF B. ZDSLMZ

ABCDEFGHIJKLMNOPQRSTUVWXYZ

189) HOL ZDNL TIM HX
VBZZ ZDFFLZZ BZ HX VBZZ
HOL XUUXNHDQBHM.

ABFHXN FOIZSLZ

---

190) YKW YAUOI YD CWYYUXC
YKUXCM VDXW UM YD FUMY
YKUXCM YD VD UX VDNTFW
DAVWA.   ADTWAY TANLFY

---

191) ADX RCWVL XEEXVAFWQE
IK DWNNFVXEE WCX:
EISXADFVR AI LI, EISXADFVR
AI QIBX, WVL EISXADFVR AI
DINX KIC.

WQQWV P. ODWQSXCE

ABCDEFGHIJKLMNOPQRSTUVWXYZ

192) JZ NMLOM DN XO
JMMOWFBIOBXFO NZO CEPD
BFTBKP XO LJVVOMOZD.

ININ IQBZOF

193) V BSLZEZIU VEEZERMU
CZTT PSE LSTIU VTT JSRK
BKSOTUDL, ORE ZE CZTT
VPPSJ UPSRXQ BUSBTU ES
DVFU ZE CSKEQ EQU UGGSKE.

QUKD VTOKZXQE

194) LHMLWH XPYC STRD
PRYHUHOYO WPNH, RMY MRWD
WMRFHOY, ZIY CTLLPHOY.

FHMUFH STYYCHX TWWHR

ABCDEFGHIJKLMNOPQRSTUVWXYZ

195) QRC PNCDQCN QRC
FBJJBKOTQW, QRC HXNC QRC
PTXNW BY IONHXOYQBYP BQ.

CMBKONOI

---

196) V MRB'E EYVBI
ZBCEYVBW VH FBSJZQVHEVG
VP CRF LJQVJAJ CRF GZB
MR VE. SVGYZSM Q. JAZBH

---

197) QBLDUGLDQ
BVVBNUSEGUZ MEBPMQ,
JSU LBQU BI UYD UGLD
GU QEDXMQ SV XET UYDE
RSGDUWZ QUDXWQ XFXZ.

TBSH WXNQBE

ABCDEFGHIJKLMNOPQRSTUVWXYZ

198) MXFAHNUT RNUT'E XRYYK
OFEX TZEXFTC EZ FCTZNU,
RTH EXRE'W OXRE YRNUTEW
OUNU MNUREUH BZN.

ZCHUT TRWX

---

199) CXBHR VXB DBMR ARRKDI
WRMRJ FJBV BDA; CXRI TEI
AZR BY BDA EFR, PNC CXRI
AZR IBNWF.

HZJ EJCXNJ KZWRJB

---

200) IQFTF UV CLAE CLF
QGXXULFVV UL AUKF, IC
ACOF GLS YF ACOFS.

WFCTWF VGLSV

ABCDEFGHIJKLMNOPQRSTUVWXYZ

201) Y BJHTP DGXXJL RL DRMG
BPYB JLG PYX BJ DGYKL RX
BPYB LJB GIGKVEJWV CRXPGX
VJH CGDD.   WYL KYBPGK

---

202) JQOBV VBXA VBXLE.
VBX'TT QJFJA MJ VBXQCJA
LEGQ VBX GAJ GL LEDP FJAV
KBKJQL.   ZEGH PXCC

---

203) W SWH INZ
LYZGYWQVDHWVJQ DH NDQ
GNZZQDHO IDAA DHJTDVWUAX
NWTJ NDQ GNZDGJ SWKJ MZY
NDS UX GDYGESQVWHGJ.
          NEHVJY Q. VNZSLQZH

ABCDEFGHIJKLMNOPQRSTUVWXYZ

204) GMXGYM ZUYY ADYR

DLXJA IXJ ZKMF AKMI MFNI IXJ

DFV AKM YUEM IXJ YMDV. YMA

AKMB. IXJ DEEMTAMV AKMUQ

YUEM. VXF'A YMA AKMB

DEEMTA IXJQC.   JFRFXZF

---

205) ID AZZK EZ FZCXNDGO.

GMNEDT EZ FZCX IZKF, EZ

FZCX BDYXE. LD'XD UDXF

BYXK ZT ZCXNDGUDN, YTK

LD'XD YGLYFN ODDGMTA GMHD

LD'XD TZE KZMTA DTZCAB.

ME'N Y EDXXMIGF BYXK PZI.

          JYXWMY LYGGYWD

ABCDEFGHIJKLMNOPQRSTUVWXYZ

206) FER SZMUWZ FERY EPW

CUMZ. SEW'J CZJ EJQZY

HZEHCZ PYUJZ FERY BAYUHJ.

EHYVQ PUWMYZF

---

207) ML SCK VCE'P WPGEV

LCX WCTIPNMEZ SCK DMYY

LGYY LCX GESPNMEZ.

TGYOCYT A

---

208) FTEI KR BC CMHEY ZTNR

KR KBQ XDFH ODCZDEV RKQ

XZDEVC OH WKBNY ZTSH DR

OH YDYE'X CMHEY ZTNR KBQ

XDFH ODCZDEV.

TNHATEYHQ OKKNNWKXX

ABCDEFGHIJKLMNOPQRSTUVWXYZ

209) SIT SZQEUEQT PHZBOHJ
ZNHSQEUH KXHI QXH YBHN
ZSNHJ SPBWQ YBEID EQ
NEDXQ, BN PHQQHN.

VBXI WFYELH

---

210) WJNQ YNRNQI EIOIKEA JK
ZPKW RBMKCA, LNR ZJARDW
JK WJN.   YQPKS RWCIQ

---

211) MECZ YZALJ, XIBZH HI
UIBL; MECZ GCLJ YZALJ,
DMCYL.   NYLQ HMYOZ

---

212) OYYV QLYNOS LQFQZ WX.

VQJJW AWQKVX

ABCDEFGHIJKLMNOPQRSTUVWXYZ

213) TPMJ ODZ HWM ARJB XD
GDIMDJM RJ XWDZCYM, ODZ
PDQM XPMO'YY WMIMICMW
HJB CM ARJB XD GDIMDJM
MYGM. HJB RX'YY CMKDIM
YRAM H TRYBSRWM.

TPDDQR LDYBCMWL

---

214) PAXW-QBOST JBRAP
WOBR BUA STHUE - STHUMHUE
STKS VBD KOA QBOSTV.

IO. QKVUA Q. IVAO

---

215) HPX IZQC FP OCCK FIC
GZN FP GC ZGKC FP OCCK
FIC RPPN.   JFCLICY NPWOO

ABCDEFGHIJKLMNOPQRSTUVWXYZ

216) IGENSKQOD IGK LKIMOLT.
OLKT XMKIG OLK IHG.

BVLQ RKIXVQ

---

217) QRPVRPS MZC'OP IZCXE
MZCS LYJJTXU, ZS TI MZC'SP
AVTJJ APYSLRTXU, DYAATZX
ARZCJE KP VRP ITSP VRYV
ESTOPA MZCS JTIP'A QZSW.

BTLRYPJ EPJJ

---

218) PZXXTPP SP RNL ASRGC,
AGSCZYT SP RNL AGLGC: SL
SP LVT XNZYGMT LN
XNRLSRZT LVGL XNZRLP.

ISRPLNR XVZYXVSCC

219) CJH TKPA YJ TKPA
EJDQONADEA OD CJHG
KZOMOYC, KDN YTAD ZA
YJHXT ADJHXT YJ QJMMJU
YTGJHXT. GJWKMCD EKGYAG

220) SQ MOPNVRV IVYJ-
MOSAMYNKMSNQX, BQ LQQB
SPNXLI JQW QSPVW UVQUYV
SPMS CQA TQAYB TMXS SQ
EV BQXV QXSQ CQAWIVYJ.

DVL OMEQS

221) KQDKW JCI MTJNKBJNM
WDQK XDK FNVDMBTY WCQJM.

ECYYC XTYKC

ABCDEFGHIJKLMNOPQRSTUVWXYZ

222) OA YLBA N VPIDNFA
IDNKV. IDLHB DP PTA DRLTF
STDLY CPS FAD DRAGA.

UPIR OLYYLTFI

---

223) FD LKZJF ZJ FD XROUEL,
FD XROUEL ZJ FD NOFVIL, FD
NOFVIL ZJ FD ED DU XILOFZUE
DULJLAW LUQALJJAG.

RLUIZ PLIEJDU

---

224) SRO GZ TRPKL TX WQKLP
QGF TRZO OQ WQ QGF TRZO,
RBRFX ZKLPSR OKER, LQ
EUOORF CMUO, HQFRBRF.

RWCUFW USTRFO

ABCDEFGHIJKLMNOPQRSTUVWXYZ

225) RCADAXF AR

GXNAQYXCGXW IQAGXHDJ.

AW COBGR GNGQJYXG'R HOJ

SQAFUWGQ OXH QGEZAQGR

NGQJ DAWWDG GXGQFJ.

COQB OCGXH

---

226) GC WKXNS TCECM NCZMT

YK VC VMZEC ZTS LZYDCTY,

DO YFCMC GCMC KTNQ AKQ

DT YFC GKMNS.

FCNCT BCNNCM

---

227) ESVC SY KBMU BMJJCZY

KBSEC NQF MXC LMISZT

QUBCX JEMZY. HQBZ ECZZQZ

ABCDEFGHIJKLMNOPQRSTUVWXYZ

228) XIANRMI PVNACAN TIFD
YFSAM UVL LHRGLA, XLQ
UVL'NA NAFJJU F UFTH RP
RD ZVAM.   WADDA YREJAN

---

229) V KRMYBF HYKTRTQZ
PZBRVG VRRTROWZ DTGG
EMZVRZ PYMZ PTMVEGZK
RAVB VBL DYBWZM WMOF.
                    HVRMTETV BZVG

---

230) IZCWS JYCO RLT WAC
WOMAR--WOE RLT JDBB
GWSC VYC PCIV IZCCQY
RLT'BB CXCA ACMACV.
            BWTACOQC H. ZCVCA

231) UYZFZ EFZ UXP UYGMOK E AZFKPM KYPRQC MZSZF NZ EMOFI EU, XYEU UYZI LEM YZQA, EMC XYEU UYZI LEMMPU.   AQEUP

---

232) QAPD QBFXZ XHNO TO HN QO APZ IB GBFYPEO DB PDDOSUD PIRDAHIE?

                    CHIGOID CPI EBEA

---

233) WOO OHTM HP WA MFLMKHYMAD. DQM YSKM MFLMKHYMADP BSG YWJM DQM RMDDMK.

          KWOLQ EWONS MYMKPSA

A B C D E F G H I J K L M N O P Q R S T U V W X Y Z

234) ZGEEQ SK ASUV B

EGPUSCJ PNBSE: SL JSFVK

QGH KGIVLNSCJ LG MG XHL

CVFVE JVLK QGH BCQZNVEV.

VEIB XGIXVPU

235) FM QSGMV QK VSKOJ

FGX QSKPLWMX LPQ QFMD

ZJMO FKO QK XOGE.

SGQR ERM LSKOJ

236) PKMCJKMG AXVYA KW

WVM VWJG MXN COKJKMG MV

SNTAKAM OBM MXN COKJKMG

MV AMCTM VPNT.

E. AQVMM EKMDUNTCJF

ABCDEFGHIJKLMNOPQRSTUVWXYZ

237) OTV KTVVDY RQWKDIGZ
VGS DKGTVW XVPGWW UG
UTW YUG KDXZTMG YD PDWG
WQMUY DA YUG WUDZG.

TVRZG MQRG

---

238) WKXFO PKX TEOZS UL
TZL ZEO AXVRJQZRW XD
SZRL WKJRVF WKZW OFAZYO
WKXFO PKX TEOZS XRGL ZW
RJVKW.   OTVZE ZGGZR YXO

---

239) NWLQL EQL ZR
PWRQNKANP NR EZS YJEKL
HRQNW XRFZX.

DLBLQJS PFJJP

ABCDEFGHIJKLMNOPQRSTUVWXYZ

240) STU GVKC YHOTS QYGUSVGUQ SY PU CVJUXSUC STBS VS GBL XUSHXK SY PUSSUX STVKIVKO. DTBUCXHQ

241) MAH OJS JPAZB VDJRZXM, IHX MAH OJSSAX JPAZB XTD OASNDUHDSODN AK JPAZBZSF VDJRZXM.   JMS VJSB

242) A UVAMY A'PH QAEGSPHXHQ UVH EHGXHU SC WACH - BSO KOEU VZMT ZXSOMQ OMUAW BSO THU OEHQ US AU.

                    GVZXWHE N. EGVOWF

83

ABCDEFGHIJKLMNOPQRSTUVWXYZ

243) IDTYSRSF YDS HOVJ CX
HTV QTV QCVQSORS, OY
QTV TQDOSRS.

I. QPSHSVY BYCVS

---

244) DKDGV BHAHUCEV CM
ET QD TKDGBTUD QV
DZNIGHZBD.   KCGXCA

---

245) GFCB GC HJKKEQ QJ
MHQEJB, QJ MHQXMZZR
PJEBN AJKCQFEBN YMQFCY
QFMB LCCZEBN QYMWWCP
VR CTCBQA, QFC AQYCAA
VCHJKCA KMBMNCMVZC.

NYCN MBPCYAJB

ABCDEFGHIJKLMNOPQRSTUVWXYZ

246) PAV'D SADTCB QFLD
DA SC SCDDCB DTRV KAFB
IAVDCHYABRBZCL AB
YBCPCICLLABL. DBK DA SC
SCDDCB DTRV KAFBLCWX.

NZWWZRH XRFWMVCB

---

247) UN YGXXHZ RNM YLQR
ENL ULZTH G FZLSFH VX
MNU'X FHX KHXXHZ.

HJGU HTGZ

---

248) YC ASAOIETYLB PAAGP
EJ XA BJYLB RAFF, IJD TUSA
JXSYJDPFI JSAOFJJVAH
PJGAETYLB. ULJLIGJDP

85

249) ISDQJLYQ GHILDT KIT
GH BX DQH HTH JE DQH
GHQJSNHW, DQH EHHSBXY JE
GHBXY GHILDBELS HCBADA
AJSHST BX DQH KBXN JE DQH
GHQHSN.   KIWDQI GHVP

---

250) ZY ZN ZAGRSYVQY JSRA
YZAT YR YZAT YR NURC IRCQ,
YR LR VCVO PO ORFSNTUJ,
VQI NZAGUO PT.

                    TZUTTQ KVIIO

---

251) WPZGZ LX MIXW VCZ
FLYZ YVG ZEKP VY IX: VIG
VJC.   ZNLKWZWIX

ABCDEFGHIJKLMNOPQRSTUVWXYZ

252) XRHZ MZRMUZ LWZ
HLCSJB XYVF EFRWRYBF
MWZMLWLESRJ TRW WLSJQ
KLQX EFLE EFZQ LWZJ'E
ZJIRQSJB ERKLQ'X XYJXFSJZ.

                    NSUUSLH TZLEFZW

---

253) VKIP LKNPCWX FKP
LFANBNPX GRNHR DYI HFC
XPBPHV.   FIWKPD RPOUIKC

---

254) EW FRDE WHV XHMUADR
OFVN EXVFHW OFAA WDSDZ
BDV EWQ IFBBDZ VNEW VND
IZEFW XDAA FV HXXMUFDR.

                    EZWHAR BAECBHO

ABCDEFGHIJKLMNOPQRSTUVWXYZ

255) WO'G MRWZQ HWDDWZQ ON HSDV SHSB OYSO QWIRG BNT GOERZQOY SZF KNHRE - WJ BNT'ER HWDDWZQ ON SPPRKO OYR PNZGRCTRZPRG NJ FNWZQ HYSO BNT HSZO ON FN.   HYNNKW QNDFMREQ

---

256) ZFDX AW JZWHYSWAQUZ EYJ XAW YCS FDMAYSW.

X. U. XRSM

---

257) LDSFDZD UNVU SFAD FX EIWUN SFZFQK VQH RIGW LDSFDA EFSS NDSO MWDVUD UND AVMU.   EFSSFVP BVPDX

ABCDEFGHIJKLMNOPQRSTUVWXYZ

258) ECYN CV Q OXNQJ KCO ZQTBQV, QTW MGL VSGLEW JSXGP QEE JSN AQCTJ GT CJ MGL ZQT.   WQTTM UQMN

---

259) HZTZWJ YZD CHJSBGFG LH DBG SZFVW TJ ELUAVJ TGLHY PZHDGHD.

VZNLE V'CUZNF

---

260) PBXS MDES WMRTMN BHA ASMDVSKBPSMN, IBXDHQ WFKS PR BLXHRTMSAQS PUS JSRJMS TUR UBYS USMJSA NRF WFLLSSA BMRHQ PUS TBN.   PSA MSYDHS

ABCDEFGHIJKLMNOPQRSTUVWXYZ

261) YMSDX VMS'W ZHDPWD
RKZZDRR, WID THDDQMY
WM YPLD GW VGUU.

SDURMS YPSQDUP

---

262) VLK BCJBSVBPK XD
LBJESP B NBC ZKZXOT EY
VLBV, YKJKOBG VEZKY XJKO,
XSK KSHXTY VLK YBZK PXXC
VLESPY DXO VLK DEOYV
VEZK.

DOEKCOEWL SEKVFYWLK

---

263) IQKBK PKFVKT VN
ZRVMTXF IK RBK NFSI ES
PKFVKHK.   SHVY

---

264) VHT WRNP R MWHFMP.
OFNP HQ GFP. PNPQV KQPRYW
FU R MWHFMP. PNPQV JFSTYP
FU R MWHFMP. YH KP HQ SHY
YH KP.   MWTMD ZRORWSFTD

---

265) PZ PI UYZ GFIH ZY TPUW
VFCCPUGII PU YMXIGODGI,
FUW PZ PI UYZ CYIIPAOG ZY
TPUW PZ GOIGBVGXG.

FNUGI XGCCOPGX

---

266) VAW XJRK BWCR
SCMROBW MJ RMSW MU
VAW SCMROBW VX VBK.

IWXBIW ZWBJCBN UACQ

ABCDEFGHIJKLMNOPQRSTUVWXYZ

267) VQZQZMQV, KQDKHQ
UPHH TFWXQ LDF ML LDFV
OBIPDGA, GDI LDFV
PGIQGIPDGA. LDF ZOL
EOYQ O EQOVI DS XDHW –
MFI AD WDQA O EOVW-
MDPHQW QXX.   FGCGDUG

---

268) NEM FMVZMN NG T
ZLVE PLCM LF NG ETHM
QGZM AMULBBLBUF NETB
MBKLBUF.   KTHM DMLBATIQ

---

269) H ELBWPR WXHBXW
QOCRF ZMLR XMLO WXPE
QBLHJCRF. NBCHR ZCDDCHJW

ABCDEFGHIJKLMNOPQRSTUVWXYZ

270) HOT RVCT WVP SCZGFT
ZXK NTYTUCZHT WVPC YGIT,
HOT RVCT HOTCT GF GX
YGIT HV NTYTUCZHT.

VSCZO EGXICTW

---

271) FNFZMOHPPR, MAYF
MHXFD EHBF SK FNFBRMVAZC.
MVF MBSOWPF TAMV
IBSEBHDMAZHMASZ AD MVHM
IFSIPF CANF OI SZ AM MSS
DSSZ. BSWFBM WBHOPM

---

272) VTAQY TACWVJP PRUAQI
WEAZYEWP VCR KBPRPW.

RGBUWRWZP

ABCDEFGHIJKLMNOPQRSTUVWXYZ

273) OUEZUBNFAIBFAEI
ANI'F FWG OUEPCGS. AF'N
FWG NECMFAEI. AF'N FWG
MIAHGUNG'N RBX EQ NBXAIL
NFEO, NCER TERI, XEM
SEHG FEE QBNF.

GCCGI TGLGIGUGN

274) OAN EAWEQM AP HOKQ
ZVD LOSS KEVMI.

KDGOPPQ HVSSAPK

275) AEN VHNJ AEJA
ALYLCCLF YVREA RNA UNAANC
VB NDLPRE AL RNA YN
AECLPRE ALHJG. YJCI JYNDH

276) GEXQYBT KR CEN NST
YHRTCGT EZ ZTYQ, HXN
QYNSTQ NST WXIBVTCN NSYN
REVTNSKCB TART KR VEQT
KVOEQNYCN NSYC ZTYQ.

VTB GYHEN

---

277) GPX NBZN EOMF ON
MBOJ, GPFJF ON YPBY
GJOYYFK? GOEEOBS UXEVSBK

---

278) EGBN GFRSHRSO BC
KFUG JBTPM OB KWBSO USM
EGUWG GFRSHRSO BC KFUG
JBTPM OB WROFG.

FUWWRVG IBWOUS

ABCDEFGHIJKLMNOPQRSTUVWXYZ

279) ISF ZFMTWU EFWEPF

QHUO HI TW SMZO IW AF

SMEEC HT ISMI ISFC MPJMCT

TFF ISF EMTI AFIIFZ ISMU HI

JMT, ISF EZFTFUI JWZTF

ISMU HI HT, MUO ISF QXIXZF

PFTT ZFTWPRFO ISMU HI

JHPP AF.   BMZGFP EMVUWP

---

280) XAWI AUM'L DU UIGAPRU

DU LTI CAMQ CDFIU AL PRL

LP HI.   IBFTDGL LPXXI

---

281) HJDT FSD FCBD

CDQFRPD HJDT HJNZW HJDT

FSD FCBD.   ONSMNB

96

ABCDEFGHIJKLMNOPQRSTUVWXYZ

282) PTKFUR NEUK GX F RGJK
YEE LGA RE BK NFX ATEB
GXYE YCKU.   QERGK LGRRKY

---

283) U CDTE HUQ DY QXOEDQM
NIO U AXXC HUQ BDOE HXQWS.
                    B. T. RDWFZY

---

284) ZSGI SK GLJI NCXACWXI
ZFCP GLPIR. RLA OCP EIZ
GLJI GLPIR, WAZ RLA OCPPLZ
EIZ GLJI ZSGI.   DSG JLFP

---

285) HGWBW VP IN PTEEWPP
JVHGNTH GKBYPGVM.
                    PNMGNERWP

ABCDEFGHIJKLMNOPQRSTUVWXYZ

286) MCPEQKP MVTEN
HIWNIWC NIW PAMXX QX IMAL
LEAA TC IMAL WGFND
GQXXWX NIW FTQKN, HIQBI
QX NIQX: NIW VMCNWKJWC
BIWMNWJ DTE.   EKOKTHK

287) IQP DVSEI OKSI VB
KYIFXN WFUP K MPSU FEX'I
DQPX RVZ'SP AVFXN FI, FI'E
DQPX RVZ SPKWFTP RVZ
DPSP.   OPIP DPXIT

288) VXG XQQ GTKM DTGP AI
OKMI DTGP, XJR XQQ GTKM
OXLJ SEXVOXCJI.   RMXUI

ABCDEFGHIJKLMNOPQRSTUVWXYZ

289) MH CNR'ID DIDK HDAE

MVGJMKDZ UC Q JRKJNGD

NK TQAAMVB, CNR LVNP

ESD HDDAMVB NH GJMKME

PNKLMVB ESKNRBS CNR.

ZK. PQCVD P. ZCDK

290) NHFJ OXNTY PXN PCFF

LCTZ RNCHR ONN MEL AEH

SNTTCWFJ MCHB NKO XNP MEL

NHY AEH RN.   O.T. YFCNO

291) PITCT JKY'P Z BTCKNY

ZYVEITCT EIN JKY'P DZBZQST

NA MNJYL WNCT PIZY IT

PIJYUK IT DZY.   ITYCV ANCM

ABCDEFGHIJKLMNOPQRSTUVWXYZ

292) COEQOCBM CE ASNSXCBQNM. MRL ISB CB VNRP MRLN FCXE.

NCTAQNX ISNS

293) OJU EHAO LEDHGOBPO OJLPS LP ZLCU LA OH ZUBGP JHT OH SLQU HRO ZHQU, BPW OH ZUO LO IHEU LP.   EHGGLU AIJTBGON

294) ASIE GJZ'H IZ SLDOJS HX DXPS HX I JHIZVJHGBB. GH'J HTS GPFSHOJ HX JHSF OF IZV JHEGQS.

IEHTOE IJTS

ABCDEFGHIJKLMNOPQRSTUVWXYZ

295) SFR ZGDHUA FQL HTZ ZGL KTQAZ ZGDHUA ZGFZ XFH GFBBLH ZT PA. HTZGDHU DA ZGL KTQAZ ZGDHU ZGFZ XFH GFBBLH ZT PA! QDXGFQR SFXG

---

296) LD'H KID DYU WIZJ DYZD MQUZRH AIF JITK, LD'H DYU TZA AIF BZQQA LD. WIF YIWDP

---

297) ES IHX KFFDLC CAD DULDFCKCEHWZ HS HCADVZ, DZLDFEKNNI WDQKCEPD HWDZ, CADW IHX WDPDV MENN FAKWQD CAD HXCFHRD.
REFAKDN GHVJKW

298) OK OI DRKKRH KS ZSSG

PCRPQ PFQ MHRMPHR KCPF

KS ZSSG DPYG PFQ HRUHRK.

　　XPYGOR XSNFRH - GRHIRR

---

299) IEPCR KEP EDYR

CQVVRRURU DI DJHIEFJZ

DJU UPJ'I WRJIFPJ NQVT

DGR TFUUFJZ IERWCRNYRC.

　　　　NDGGH TFJZ

---

300) PMH OIMBQ PMHD

JDVGS AWVR PMH GIIMA

PMHD EVGD KM XDMA

OTXXVD KWGR PMHD EGTKW.

　　SGDP SGRTR SMDDTLLVP

ABCDEFGHIJKLMNOPQRSTUVWXYZ

301) WOG UBIN BX QJXC

YGJYTGJN EWG SGTCBCONJ

FKJI BCX WYJI VOXC TX CKJ

ROY BX QJXC YGJYTGJN EWG

EBDDBIS FKJI BC'X JUYCP.

                    HJUUP IWDT

302) SAGQW FAG SAYMI YS

YQ ZWKCYQQYUXW SG SWXX

FAYSW XYWQ QGGM DKGF

TGXGK-UXYMN.

              JRQSYM G'CJXXWP

303) MDQT DK GCT POECF,

KUTTL KGCP KG KLEOL LAT

ZVKDW.   OGCEMF OTEPEC

304) R GCIPVJTAQ VJKDW CK CXH LHGGTPTGC TG R GCHLLTAQ-GCKAH CK CXH KLCTPTGC.

HJHRAKF FKKGHEHJC

---

305) XQSETDHID SB ENZC JW MSWWJYTD JW CND YDIJQQJQI SB NZMMJQDWW.

IDSFID WZQCZLZQZ

---

306) LX WMQQJU DOMQ PXRU OJMUQMTOJ WMP CJ, FMRVOELV OJFHB PXR GXUVJQ EQ GXU M GJD BJTXLZB. UJZ BIJFQXL

ABCDEFGHIJKLMNOPQRSTUVWXYZ

307) TGGTSWZBKWU KY SVSO,
VBF V DKYO XVB DKQQ BOPOS
QOW KW JT AU NKX.

AVUVSF WVUQTS

---

308) XGITJWY JU HWG HC PXG
AHBZ'U CJFG UGWUGU. ARP
QJUPGWJWY JU IW ITP.

CTIWS PZYGT

---

309) DZ ORJ BJZO PDWJ FZ
LFXY SYKDM IFMOYFBP ORJ
YDVRO PDWJ FZ LFXY SFWL,
ORJM FMBL BJZO RKMWJW
HJFHBJ KYJ DM ORJDY
YDVRO QDMW.   XMGMFAM

ABCDEFGHIJKLMNOPQRSTUVWXYZ

310) UFFSZRYULYHT YO U
QHTXZSBMI LWYTK: YL
VUJZO QWUL YO ZDRZIIZTL
YT HLWZSO AZIHTK LH MO
UO QZII.   GHILUYSZ

---

311) CE UE GADFAJ REL
UGA NBKYDUA, GABB REL
UGA NEYQDJZ.   YDLS UHDKJ

---

312) L'N WUZQCW TC
UHMVC UVN FLXQ L FCWC
FLZQ XMYCMVC ZQUV ZM TC
FLZQ XMYCMVC UVN FLXQ L
FCWC UHMVC.

                    CWLAU UHHCVNC

A B C D E F G H I J K L M N O P Q R S T U V W X Y Z

313) AG SWSJOLBACV AX SZXO LQ VSL, KS KAEE CSWSJ ZTTJSHAZLS ZCF PS TJQYF QG KBZL KS BZWS.   NZJM ZNSCF

314) BXJVJ IVJ PE HYJJU FOGOBH EP BXJ VEIU BE JKMJFFJPMJ.   VOMXIVU WIMX

315) D NDO XG OFZ FVH QOZXV IULIUZG ZDMU ZTU JVDBU FE HIUDNG.

SFTO WDIICNFIU

316) UFO LDOOUOLU LIQBG IR PTT JL CWPJLO.   NOBICFIB

ABCDEFGHIJKLMNOPQRSTUVWXYZ

317) SP SH IBP PDU
HPQBIMUHP BK PDU HTUGSUH
PDXP HAQLSLUH, IBQ PDU
RBHP SIPUFFSMUIP, VAP PDU
BIU RBHP QUHTBIHSLU PB
GDXIMU.   GDXQFUH WXQESI

---

318) CKNH IOBP EB ORTOCB
CKNH IOBP. WJWM EU CKN
UKHDWP EP, EP HWQWQAWHB
CKN.   BOHOS ZWBBWM

---

319) RI RLT'I SWDPD CJV
OUQD BPJQ, RIL SWDPD
CJV'PD KJRTK IWUI OJVTIL.
            DFFU BRINKDPUFA

A B C D E F G H I J K L M N O P Q R S T U V W X Y Z

320) VI XGDU OIA'TH
WDYYFIEDUH DJIAU.

QDLHO LGDJHTU

---

321) VKS WRI IYNYP TY SCJYZ
FMZU ZUY CYKCBY FUK
QKPWYG VKS MIZK VKSP
GPYRE KP SC UMXUYP.

ZYPPV CYPPV

---

322) RMZ KMB'J VJMF
HDZAONBA TPGDZVP RMZ
AXMY MHK. RMZ AXMY MHK
TPGDZVP RMZ VJMF
HDZAONBA.

QNGODPH FXNJGODXK

ABCDEFGHIJKLMNOPQRSTUVWXYZ

323) T IXLGM HLNK FEDKZF KEPZ FZUFZDO EWXLD JXD MXTJU IKED QZXQGZ OETM, DKEJ FZUFZDDTJU JXD MXTJU IKED HV KZEFD GZM HZ DX EJM IXJMZFTJU IKED GTAZ KEM WZZJ GTSZ TA T'M YLOD WZZJ HVOZGA.

WFTDDEJV FZJZZ

324) MNLNG BRLN TX EM QSFP KET GNFCCK QFMP PE ZE. PSN XNGAEM QRPS ORB ZGNFIA RA IEGN XEQNGJTC PSFM EMN QRPS FCC PSN JFHPA.   TMWMEQM

CLUE ONE

1. O = S	19. K = R	37. M = N	55. R = F
2. Q = R	20. I = L	38. L = S	56. I = L
3. Z = M	21. F = N	39. N = C	57. S = R
4. A = F	22. V = B	40. X = D	58. V = L
5. Y = C	23. E = K	41. T = S	59. T = R
6. C = L	24. X = N	42. P = C	60. O = N
7. U = R	25. M = R	43. V = N	61. K = L
8. E = B	26. W = R	44. T = R	62. L = R
9. H = M	27. K = C	45. D = S	63. S = D
10. T = M	28. M = D	46. C = D	64. J = T
11. H = L	29. J = S	47. G = L	65. V = S
12. Z = R	30. I = P	48. C = S	66. F = B
13. V = M	31. X = R	49. A = N	67. M = D
14. H = S	32. T = W	50. I = C	68. R = S
15. V = L	33. H = C	51. V = L	69. U = N
16. I = D	34. Q = D	52. A = N	70. I = L
17. J = L	35. D = S	53. Z = M	71. Z = S
18. E = S	36. A = R	54. M = S	72. K = L

73. Q = N	91. V = L	109. T = C	127. L = G
74. N = M	92. Y = R	110. B = F	128. T = N
75. V = D	93. N = S	111. X = S	129. E = M
76. Z = S	94. Q = R	112. V = N	130. H = G
77. E = N	95. V = W	113. I = M	131. Q = L
78. G = R	96. W = R	114. Y = R	132. B = D
79. L = S	97. L = C	115. F = N	133. F = L
80. D = U	98. I = R	116. R = M	134. M = R
81. B = L	99. W = L	117. L = N	135. Z = G
82. J = R	100. D = S	118. E = B	136. A = S
83. L = H	101. U = N	119. Z = W	137. H = C
84. S = N	102. B = L	120. G = S	138. V = H
85. Q = D	103. S = M	121. C = D	139. T = R
86. A = K	104. O = G	122. N = M	140. I = N
87. E = S	105. K = T	123. O = N	141. A = S
88. X = N	106. C = N	124. D = G	142. Q = P
89. D = S	107. L = M	125. W = L	143. L = D
90. A = N	108. O = J	126. K = P	144. G = M

145. A = N	163. F = D	181. E = C	199. A = D
146. B = M	164. W = N	182. N = W	200. L = N
147. T = S	165. M = R	183. S = D	201. W = D
148. N = L	166. O = M	184. G = K	202. V = Y
149. D = C	167. W = C	185. R = M	203. L = P
150. W = R	168. A = W	186. B = V	204. Y = L
151. P = F	169. L = P	187. R = M	205. L = W
152. L = N	170. H = G	188. Z = R	206. Y = R
153. K = N	171. E = N	189. N = R	207. T = M
154. A = M	172. T = F	190. V = D	208. O = W
155. O = S	173. W = N	191. Q = L	209. Z = C
156. G = M	174. F = W	192. I = C	210. R = T
157. F = H	175. E = N	193. D = M	211. M = W
158. X = L	176. Z = C	194. R = N	212. V = D
159. H = F	177. H = V	195. N = R	213. T = W
160. T = M	178. X = D	196. B = N	214. O = R
161. C = L	179. N = P	197. Q = S	215. N = D
162. O = W	180. A = L	198. M = C	216. X = C

217. J = L	235. S = R	253. B = L	271. B = R
218. X = C	236. A = S	254. W = N	272. P = S
219. G = R	237. V = N	255. H = W	273. T = N
220. O = C	238. T = D	256. X = H	274. K = S
221. Y = N	239. P = S	257. S = L	275. Y = M
222. I = S	240. K = N	258. T = N	276. G = C
223. X = C	241. M = Y	259. V = L	277. E = L
224. S = L	242. G = C	260. N = Y	278. F = H
225. C = M	243. H = M	261. Y = M	279. P = L
226. N = L	244. G = R	262. S = N	280. C = M
227. Z = N	245. N = G	263. P = B	281. S = R
228. X = C	246. V = N	264. M = C	282. R = S
229. P = M	247. Z = R	265. C = P	283. B = W
230. A = R	248. F = L	266. B = R	284. J = R
231. X = W	249. K = M	267. M = B	285. P = C
232. E = G	250. Q = N	268. B = N	286. C = R
233. Y = M	251. X = S	269. W = S	287. D = W
234. P = C	252. W = R	270. R = M	288. O = P

289. K = R	298. H = R	307. A = B	316. C = P
290. H = N	299. N = L	308. W = N	317. H = S
291. C = R	300. S = M	309. B = L	318. H = R
292. X = D	301. I = N	310. S = R	319. F = L
293. E = M	302. C = M	311. N = C	320. L = C
294. J = S	303. O = R	312. W = R	321. P = R
295. S = B	304. L = P	313. F = D	322. F = P
296. W = L	305. I = G	314. V = R	323. J = N
297. F = C	306. B = S	315. N = M	324. Q = W

CLUE TWO

1. H = M	19. G = P	37. X = G	55. E = R
2. V = Y	20. M = R	38. E = N	56. K = N
3. F = W	21. G = L	39. Q = N	57. L = M
4. Z = R	22. L = C	40. K = C	58. O = F
5. Z = B	23. Y = N	41. M = Y	59. C = S
6. K = M	24. D = S	42. B = N	60. E = A
7. Y = D	25. J = S	43. H = L	61. P = N
8. S = R	26. A = P	44. A = D	62. N = F
9. P = S	27. A = R	45. J = C	63. Y = S
10. R = G	28. G = R	46. E = C	64. Z = N
11. F = G	29. T = D	47. F = P	65. O = R
12. A = N	30. H = R	48. Z = R	66. V = R
13. K = W	31. C = S	49. I = S	67. J = N
14. A = D	32. E = B	50. K = L	68. Y = D
15. M = C	33. C = R	51. A = N	69. X = S
16. Q = R	34. R = L	52. P = R	70. O = C
17. X = S	35. E = W	53. B = L	71. N = R
18. M = C	36. H = S	54. C = M	72. G = C

73. X = L	91. K = C	109. U = L	127. O = N
74. X = C	92. C = L	110. J = R	128. W = P
75. T = R	93. T = A	111. M = D	129. F = R
76. O = D	94. R = N	112. N = T	130. C = H
77. J = S	95. W = R	113. B = L	131. Y = N
78. S = G	96. T = D	114. H = N	132. O = M
79. U = R	97. R = D	115. I = L	133. D = R
80. V = C	98. L = M	116. E = N	134. T = G
81. F = M	99. M = S	117. O = M	135. F = R
82. W = S	100. F = L	118. T = C	136. L = P
83. G = N	101. Y = T	119. K = B	137. L = N
84. U = D	102. X = S	120. A = N	138. E = F
85. W = S	103. H = L	121. D = L	139. B = M
86. M = R	104. J = R	122. S = R	140. L = R
87. L = D	105. E = L	123. S = V	141. R = N
88. K = M	106. L = S	124. X = D	142. P = M
89. W = M	107. Q = N	125. Z = G	143. X = S
90. Y = L	108. E = C	126. B = R	144. D = R

145. Z = M	163. H = N	181. Q = N	199. D = L
146. D = C	164. Q = M	182. A = B	200. V = S
147. Z = M	165. S = B	183. R = M	201. X = S
148. J = R	166. K = P	184. T = F	202. C = G
149. S = N	167. G = M	185. O = L	203. G = C
150. B = L	168. Y = R	186. V = N	204. E = F
151. L = M	169. U = C	187. L = G	205. K = D
152. V = P	170. C = N	188. C = W	206. P = W
153. G = M	171. Y = G	189. Z = S	207. Y = L
154. L = R	172. E = D	190. A = R	208. X = T
155. Y = D	173. L = G	191. V = N	209. I = N
156. L = N	174. A = N	192. F = L	210. W = Y
157. V = M	175. I = W	193. B = P	211. Z = N
158. V = N	176. K = L	194. W = L	212. X = S
159. B = S	177. J = Y	195. P = G	213. B = D
160. S = R	178. G = N	196. Q = L	214. Q = W
161. J = C	179. Z = L	197. E = N	215. I = H
162. B = K	180. E = D	198. H = D	216. G = R

217. S = R	235. O = W	253. K = R	271. P = L
218. A = F	236. J = L	254. A = L	272. W = T
219. M = L	237. W = S	255. K = P	273. N = S
220. L = G	238. R = N	256. S = N	274. E = H
221. Q = R	239. Q = R	257. L = B	275. H = D
222. Y = L	240. X = R	258. M = Y	276. V = M
223. U = N	241. V = R	259. H = N	277. G = W
224. F = R	242. W = L	260. M = L	278. W = R
225. X = N	243. V = N	261. S = N	279. U = S
226. M = R	244. B = C	262. Z = M	280. F = K
227. E = L	245. Y = R	263. F = L	281. C = B
228. Y = M	246. B = R	264. N = V	282. Y = T
229. B = N	247. U = N	265. U = N	283. C = R
230. Z = P	248. P = S	266. R = L	284. G = M
231. Q = L	249. G = B	267. V = R	285. M = P
232. I = N	250. A = M	268. A = B	286. P = G
233. K = R	251. N = P	269. B = R	287. X = N
234. I = M	252. J = N	270. C = R	288. G = Y

289. P = W	298. I = S	307. W = T	316. B = N
290. F = L	299. T = K	308. U = S	317. Q = R
291. V = Y	300. D = R	309. W = D	318. B = S
292. N = R	301. U = M	310. I = L	319. O = C
293. A = S	302. Q = S	311. Y = M	320. U = T
294. D = C	303. Z = M	312. F = W	321. W = C
295. Q = R	304. F = R	313. J = R	322. T = B
296. A = Y	305. W = S	314. F = L	323. F = R
297. R = M	306. L = N	315. I = R	324. A = S

SOLUTIONS

1) A goal is not always meant to be reached, it often serves simply as something to aim at.   Bruce Lee

2) Breathe. Let go. And remind yourself that this very moment is the only one you know you have for sure.
Oprah Winfrey

3) Too much of a good thing can be wonderful.
Mae West

4) Failure is simply the opportunity to begin again, this time more intelligently.   Henry Ford

5) It's always the little decisions that have the biggest impact.   Mark Cuban

6) The only way of finding the limits of the possible is by going beyond them into the impossible.
Arthur C. Clarke

7) If you don't think every day is a good day, just try missing one.   Cavett Robert

8) Don't expect not to be afraid. Real courage is being scared to death and going ahead anyway.
Brett Wilson

9) Nothing builds self-esteem and self-confidence like accomplishment.   Thomas Carlyle

10) Making mistakes simply means you are learning
faster.   Weston H. Agor

11) Laughter is a tranquilizer with no side effects.
                                    Arnold H. Glasgow

12) Let us not be content to wait and see what will
happen, but give us the determination to make the
right things happen.   Horace Mann

13) If you want to make your dreams come true, the
first thing you have to do is wake up.   J.M. Power

14) Those who say it can't be done are usually
interrupted by others doing it.   James A. Baldwin

15) If you blithely do what you do and you're good at
what you do, and try to be a decent person, you can
succeed.   Michael Patrick Jann

16) The thing you have to be prepared for is that
other people don't always dream your dream.
                                    Linda Ronstadt

17) A smile is a curve that sets everything straight.
                                    Phyllis Diller

18) Much of the stress that people feel doesn't come
from having too much to do. It comes from not
finishing what they started.   David Allen

19) Never tell people how to do things. Tell them what to do and they will surprise you with their ingenuity.   George S. Patton

20) Through humor, you can soften some of the worst blows that life delivers. And once you find laughter, no matter how painful your situation might be, you can survive it.   Bill Cosby

21) You don't need anybody to tell you who you are or what you are. You are what you are!
                    John Lennon

22) Nothing stops the man who desires to achieve. Every obstacle is simply a course to develop his achievement muscle. It's a strengthening of his powers of accomplishment.   Eric Butterworth

23) If you only do what you know you can do- you never do very much.   Tom Krause

24) Once you replace negative thoughts with positive ones, you'll start having positive results.
                    Willie Nelson

25) The happiness of your life depends upon the quality of your thoughts; therefore guard accordingly.
                    Marcus Aurelius

26) A pinch of probability is worth a pound of perhaps.   James Thurber

27) Every person, all the events of your life are there because you have drawn them there. What you choose to do with them is up to you.   Richard Bach

28) You have to risk going too far to discover just how far you can really go.   Drake

29) The way to get started is to quit talking and begin doing.   Walt Disney

30) Small deeds done are better than great deeds planned.   Peter Marshall

31) Reach high, for stars lie hidden in your soul. Dream deep, for every dream precedes the goal.
Pamela Vaull Starr

32) You can always become better.   Tiger Woods

33) You don't develop courage by being happy in your relationships everyday. You develop it by surviving difficult times and challenging adversity.
Epicurus

34) You don't need water to feel like you're drowning, do you?   Jodi Picoult

35) When we put a limit on what we will do, we put a limit on what we can do.   Charles Schwab

36) The greatest thief this world has ever produced is procrastination, and he is still at large.

Henry Wheelter Shaw

37) To think too long about doing a thing often becomes its undoing.

Eva Young

38) One of the greatest labor-saving inventions of today is tomorrow.

Vincent T. Foss

39) To accomplish great things, we must not only act, but also dream; not only plan, but also believe.

Anatole France

40) Not everything that is faced can be changed, but nothing can be changed until it is faced.

James A. Baldwin

41) May all your troubles last as long as your New Year's resolutions.

Joey Adams

42) Preconceived notions are the locks on the door to wisdom.

Merry Browne

43) To expect life to treat you good is foolish as hoping a bull won't hit you because you are a vegetarian.

Rosanne Barr

44) Always behave like a duck- keep calm and unruffled on the surface, but paddle like the devil underneath.

Jacob M. Braude

45) Success is a state of mind. If you want success, start thinking of yourself as a success.

Dr. Joyce Brothers

46) Take a chance! All life is a chance. The man who goes the furthest is generally the one who is willing to do and dare. Dale Carnegie

47) You are what you believe yourself to be.

Paulo Coelho

48) Know the true value of time; snatch, seize, and enjoy every moment of it. No idleness, no delay, no procrastination; never put off till tomorrow what you can do today. Lord Chesterfield

49) To keep your marriage brimming, with love in the wedding cup, whenever you're wrong, admit it; whenever you're right, shut up. Ogden Nash

50) If you spent your life concentrating on what everyone else thought of you, would you forget who you really were? Jodi Picoult

51) Only you can judge your life. You have to live up to your own expectations. Wolfgang Puck

52) Let fear be a counselor and not a jailer.

Anthony Robbins

53) To make mistakes is human; to stumble is commonplace; to be able to laugh at yourself is maturity. William A. Ward

54) Strength does not come from physical capacity. It comes from an indomitable will. Mahatma Gandhi

55) People love others not for who they are but for how they make them feel. Irwin Federman

56) A little lie is like a little pregnancy it doesn't take long before everyone knows. C. S. Lewis

57) Success means having the courage, the determination, and the will to become the person you believe you were meant to be. George Sheehan

58) The first duty of love is to listen. Paul Tillich

59) When you've seen beyond yourself, then you may find, peace of mind is waiting there.
George Harrison

60) Everything you do prepares you for the next thing. John Abel

61) What a pity human beings can't exchange problems. Everyone knows exactly how to solve the other fellow's. Olin Miller

62) I've been absolutely terrified every moment of my life - and I've never let it keep me from doing a single thing I wanted to do.　　　　　　Georgia O'Keeffe

63) Do not let yesterdays disappointments overshadow on tomorrows dreams because your life is like a mirror, if you keep smiling it smiles right back at you…So, keep smiling.　　　　　　Unknown

64) There is no evidence that the tongue is connected to the brain.　　　　　　Frank Tyger

65) Success is to be measured not so much by the position that one has reached in life as by the obstacles which he has overcome.
　　　　　　Booker T. Washington

66) The biggest risk you can take is to take no risk.
　　　　　　Mark Zuckerberg

67) The three great essentials to achieve anything worth while are, first, hard work; second, stick-to-itiveness; third, common sense.　　　Thomas Edison

68) Our lives are a sum total of the choices we have made.　　　　　　Dr. Wayne W. Dyer

69) Nothing has more strength than dire necessity.
　　　　　　Epictetus

70) Whatever course you decide upon, there is always someone to tell you that you are wrong. There are always difficulties arising, which tempt you to believe that your critics are right. To map out a course of action and follow it to an end requires courage.   Ralph Waldo Emerson

71) To desire is to obtain; to aspire is to achieve.
                                                        James Allen

72) Excellence is not a singular act, but a habit. You are what you repeatedly do.   Shaquille O'Neal

73) Doing nothing is very hard to do…you never know when you're finished.   Leslie Nielsen

74) Patience is something you admire in the driver behind you, and scorn in the one ahead.
                                                        Mac McCleary

75) A compromise is the art of dividing a cake in such a way that everyone believes he has the biggest piece.   Ludwig Erhard

76) It is not because things are difficult that we do not dare, it is because we do not dare that they are difficult.   Seneca

77) Success is dependent on effort.   Sophocles

78) The big secret in life is that there is no big secret. Whatever your goal, you can get there if you're willing to work.   Oprah Winfrey

79) Experience is the only school from which no one ever graduates.   Evan Esar

80) The most called-upon prerequisite of a friend is an accessible ear.   Maya Angelou

81) All problems become smaller if you don't dodge them but confront them.   William F. Halsey

82) It is important that you recognize your progress and take pride in your accomplishments. Share your achievements with others. Brag a little. The recognition and support of those around you is nurturing.   Rosemarie Rossetti

83) One needs something to believe in, something for which one can have whole-hearted enthusiasm. One needs to feel that one's life has meaning, that one is needed in this world.   Hannah Senesh

84) When two people decide to get a divorce, it isn't a sign that they "don't understand" one another, but a sign that they have, at last, begun to.
                    Helen Rowland

85) If there are things you don't like in the world you grew up in, make your own life different.
                    Dave Thomas

86) Learn to listen. Opportunity could be knocking at your door very softly.   Frank Tyger

87) Set out each day believing in your dreams. Know without a doubt that you were made for amazing things.   Josh Hinds

88) You must get involved to have an impact. No one is impressed with the won – lost record of the referee.   John H. Holcomb

89) My favorite things in life don't cost any money. It's really clear that the most precious resource we all have is time.   Steve Jobs

90) You will never win if you never begin.   Helen Rowland

91) Life is like a ten-speed bicycle. Most of us have gears we never use.   Charles M. Schulz

92) You find peace not by rearranging the circumstances of your life, but by realizing who you are at the deepest level.   Eckhart Tolle

93) Seven days without laughter make one weak.   Joel Goodman

94) English is a funny language. That explains why we park our car on the driveway and drive our car on the parkway.   Mark Grasso

95) We never know the worth of water till the well is dry.   Thomas Fuller

96) You are never too old to set another goal or to dream a new dream.   Les Brown

97) It's the constant and determined effort that breaks down all resistance, sweeps away all obstacles.
Claude M. Bristol

98) All changes are more or less tinged with melancholy, for what we are leaving behind is part of ourselves.   Amelia Barr

99) Life is the sum of all your choices.   Albert Camus

100) The most unfortunate thing that happens to a person who fears failure is that he limits himself by becoming afraid to try anything new.   Leo Buscaglia

101) When you start to develop your powers of empathy and imagination, the whole world opens up to you.   Susan Sarandon

102) A joy shared is a joy doubled.   C. S. Lewis

103) Waste your money and you're only out of money, but waste your time and you've lost a part of your life.   Michael LeBoeuf

104) Don't try to figure out what other people want to hear from you; figure out what you have to say.
Barbara Kingsolver

105) Tell the truth, or someone will tell it for you.
Stephanie Klein

106) To begin to think with purpose is to enter the ranks of those strong ones who only recognize failure as one of the pathways to attainment.   James Allen

107) You must love yourself before you love another. By accepting yourself and fully being what you are, your simple presence can make others happy.
Mignon McLaughlin

108) In today's rush we all think too much, seek too much, want too much and forget about the joy of just Being.   Eckhart Tolle

109) Count the garden by the flowers, never by the leaves that fall. Count your life with smiles and not the tears that roll.   Unknown

110) The future is an opportunity.   J. F. Ware

111) The surest way to escape anxiety and defeat despair is action. Do, don't dwell.
Michael Josephson

112) Death is nothing, but to live defeated and inglorious is to die daily.   Napoleon Bonaparte

113) The greatest mistake you can make in life is to continually be afraid you will make one.

Elbert Hubbard

114) The most important story we'll ever write in life is our own-not with ink, but with our daily choices.

Richard Paul Evans

115) I really don't think life is about the I-could-have-beens. Life is only about the I-tried-to-do. I don't mind the failure but I can't imagine that I'd forgive myself if I didn't try.

Nikki Giovanni

116) Human beings, by changing the inner attitudes of their minds, can change the outer aspects of their lives.

William James

117) On some days you get what you want, and on others, you get what you need.

Hunter S. Thompson

118) There's no fool like an old fool - you can't beat experience.

Jacob M. Braude

119) The best way to convince a fool that he is wrong is to let him have his own way.

Josh Billings

120) The willingness to accept responsibility for one's own life is the source from which self-respect springs.

Joan Didion

121) Anything you really want, you can attain, if you really go after it. Dr. Wayne W. Dyer

122) The dread of doing a task uses up more time and energy than doing the task itself. Rita Emmett

123) Winners never quit, and quitters never win.
Vince Lombardi

124) He who labors diligently need never despair; for all things are accomplished by diligence and labor.
Menander

125) People with goals succeed because they know where they're going. Earl Nightingale

126) You can either complain or look for opportunity in every problem. I prefer opportunity. Paul Orfalea

127) Take calculated risks. That is quite different from being rash. George S. Patton

128) We are what we pretend to be, so we must be careful about what we pretend to be.
Kurt Vonnegut

129) You must first be who you really are, then do what you need to do, in order to have what you want. Margaret Young

130) Nothing great was ever achieved without enthusiasm. William Wrigley Jr.

131) You don't have to see the whole staircase, just take the first step.   Martin Luther King, Jr.

132) You may be deceived if you trust too much, but you will live in torment if you do not trust enough.
                                         Frank Crane

133) Trust only movement. Life happens at the level of events, not of words. Trust movement.
                                         Alfred Adler

134) If you doubt you can accomplish something, then you can't accomplish it. You have to have confidence in your ability, and then be tough enough to follow through.   Rosalyn Carter

135) Whatever you're going through in your life, don't ever give up.   Mariah Carey

136) A person can't change all at once.
                                         Stephen King

137) Find joy in everything you choose to do. Every job, relationship, home...it's your responsibility to love it, or change it.   Chuck Palahniuk

138) All marriages are happy. It's living together afterwards that is difficult.   Unknown

139) All glory comes from daring to begin.
                                   Eugene F. Ware

140) If only we'd stop trying to be happy we could have a pretty good time. 　　　　Edith Wharton

141) All things happen for a reason, even though it's an eternity sometimes before we learn those reasons. 　　　　Unknown

142) Love never fails. Character never quits. And with patience and persistence, dreams do come true. 　　　　Pete Maravich

143) I never dreamed about success. I worked for it. 　　　　Estee Lauder

144) Smart people know their strengths, but happy people are the ones who have accepted their flaws. 　　　　Kimo

145) If you'll not settle for anything less than your best, you will be amazed at what you can accomplish in your lives. 　　　　Vince Lombardi

146) Success seems to be connected to action. Successful people keep moving. They make mistakes, but they never quit. 　　J. Willard Marriott

147) Friendship is like money, easier made than kept. 　　　　Samuel Butler

148) Nothing is more despicable than respect based on fear. 　　　　Albert Camus

149) Success is more permanent when you achieve it without destroying your principles.   Walter Cronkite

150) Never interrupt someone doing what you said couldn't be done.   Amelia Earhart

151) There comes a time in the affairs of man when he must take the bull by the tail and face the situation.   W. C. Fields

152) A happy person is not a person in a certain set of circumstances, but rather a person with a certain set of attitudes.   Hugh Downs

153) The natural flights of the human mind are not from pleasure to pleasure but from hope to hope.
                          Samuel Johnson

154) Life isn't a matter of milestones, but of moments.
                          Rose Kennedy

155) Accepting all the good and bad about someone. It's a great thing to aspire to. The hard part is actually doing it.   Sarah Dessen

156) One never notices what has been done; one can only see what remains to be done.   Marie Curie

157) Why are some of the best things in life some of the things that hurt us the most?   Amy Davis

158) You never fail until you stop trying.

Albert Einstein

159) Face your fears and doubts, and new worlds will open to you.   Robert Kiyosaki

160) A year from now you may wish you had started today.   Karen Lamb

161) Knowledge will give you power, but character respect.   Bruce Lee

162) When life knocks you down you have two choices - stay down or get up.   Tom Krause

163) There is only one person who could ever make you happy, and that person is you.   David Burns

164) Life's not about the people who act to your face. It's about the people who remain true behind your back.   Anonymous

165) The bond that links your true family is not one of blood, but of respect and joy in each other's life.

Richard Bach

166) Opportunities to find deeper powers within ourselves come when life seems most challenging.

Joseph Campbell

167) The most important thing in communication is hearing what isn't said.   Peter Drucker

168) How people treat you is their karma. How you react is yours.   Dr. Wayne W. Dyer

169) It is not so much our friend's help that helps us as the confidence of their help.   Epicurus

170) People often say that motivation doesn't last. Well, neither does bathing - that's why we recommend it daily.   Zig Ziglar

171) Focus on the journey, not the destination. Joy is found not in finishing an activity but in doing it.
                    Greg Anderson

172) Failure is not to be feared. It is from failure that most growth comes.   Dee Hock

173) They say that love is more important than money, but have you ever tried to pay your bills with a hug?   Anonymous

174) As you walk down the fairway of life you must smell the roses, for you only get to play one round.
                    Ben Hogan

175) If you do what you've always done, you'll get what you've always gotten.   Anthony Robbins

176) True love comes quietly, without banners or flashing lights. If you hear bells, get your ears checked.   Erich Segal

177) Striving for success without hard work is like trying to harvest where you haven't planted.

David Bly

178) An idea that is developed and put into action is more important than an idea that exists only as an idea.

Buddha

179) It's the simple things in life that are the most extraordinary.

Paulo Coelho

180) Life is like a coin. You can spend it any way you wish, but you only spend it once.

Lillian Dickson

181) Not everything that can be counted counts, and not everything that counts can be counted.

Albert Einstein

182) Know and believe in yourself, and what others think won't disturb you.

William Feather

183) Freedom is not worth having if it does not include the freedom to make mistakes.

Mahatma Gandhi

184) We should not let our fears hold us back from pursuing our hopes.

John F. Kennedy

185) It takes as much courage to have tried and failed as it does to have tried and succeeded.

Anne Morrow Lindbergh

186) Winning isn't everything, but wanting to win is.
Vince Lombardi

187) There are so many things that we wish we had done yesterday, so few that we feel like doing today.
Mignon McLaughlin

188) Reality isn't the way you wish things to be, nor the way they appear to be, but the way they actually are.
Robert J. Ringer

189) The sure way to miss success is to miss the opportunity.
Victor Chasles

190) The trick to getting things done is to list things to do in doable order.
Robert Brault

191) The grand essentials of happiness are: something to do, something to love, and something to hope for.
Allan K. Chalmers

192) In order to be irreplaceable one must always be different.
Coco Chanel

193) A positive attitude will not solve all your problems, but it will annoy enough people to make it worth the effort.
Herm Albright

194) People with many interests live, not only longest, but happiest.
George Matthew Allen

195) The greater the difficulty, the more the glory in surmounting it.   Epicurus

196) I don't think anything is unrealistic if you believe you can do it.   Richard L. Evans

197) Sometimes opportunity knocks, but most of the time it sneaks up and then quietly steals away.
                                                    Doug Larson

198) Children aren't happy with nothing to ignore, and that's what parents were created for.
                                                    Ogden Nash

199) Those who love deeply never grow old; they may die of old age, but they die young.
                                              Sir Arthur Pinero

200) There is only one happiness in life, to love and be loved.   George Sands

201) A tough lesson in life that one has to learn is that not everybody wishes you well.   Dan Rather

202) Enjoy your youth. You'll never be younger than you are at this very moment.   Chad Sugg

203) A man who procrastinates in his choosing will inevitably have his choice made for him by circumstance.   Hunter S. Thompson

204) People will talk about you when they envy you and the life you lead. Let them. You affected their life. Don't let them affect yours.   Unknown

205) Be good to yourself. Listen to your body, to your heart. We're very hard on ourselves, and we're always feeling like we're not doing enough. It's a terribly hard job.   Marcia Wallace

206) You define your own life. Don't let other people write your script.   Oprah Winfrey

207) If you don't stand for something you will fall for anything.   Malcolm X

208) Many of us spend half of our time wishing for things we could have if we didn't spend half our time wishing.   Alexander Woollcott

209) Any activity becomes creative when the doer cares about doing it right, or better.   John Updike

210) Your future depends on many things, but mostly on you.   Frank Tyger

211) When angry, count to four; when very angry, swear.   Mark Twain

212) Good enough never is.   Debbi Fields

213) When you are kind to someone in trouble, you hope they'll remember and be kind to someone else. And it'll become like a wildfire.   Whoopi Goldberg

214) Self-worth comes from one thing - thinking that you are worthy.   Dr. Wayne W. Dyer

215) You have to feel the bad to be able to feel the good.   Stephen Dorff

216) Arguments are healthy. They clear the air.
                                        John Deacon

217) Whether you've found your calling, or if you're still searching, passion should be the fire that drives your life's work.   Michael Dell

218) Success is not final, failure is not fatal: it is the courage to continue that counts.   Winston Churchill

219) You have to have confidence in your ability, and then be tough enough to follow through.
                                        Rosalyn Carter

220) To achieve self-actualization, do good things for other people that you would want to be done onto yourself.   Meg Cabot

221) Truth may sometimes hurt but delusion harms.
                                        Vanna Bonta

222) Be like a postage stamp. Stick to one thing until you get there.   Josh Billings

223) To exist is to change, to change is to mature, to mature is to go on creating oneself endlessly.
                                    Henri Bergson

224) Let us begin by doing our best to do our best, every single time, no matter what, forever.
                                    Edward Albert

225) Smiling is environment friendly. It makes everyone's day brighter and requires very little energy.   Mark Amend

226) We could never learn to be brave and patient, if there were only joy in the world.   Helen Keller

227) Life is what happens while you are making other plans.   John Lennon

228) Cherish forever what makes you unique, cuz you're really a yawn if it goes.   Bette Midler

229) A strong positive mental attitude will create more miracles than any wonder drug.   Patricia Neal

230) Speak when you are angry--and you will make the best speech you'll ever regret.
                                    Laurence J. Peter

231) There are two things a person should never be angry at, what they can help, and what they cannot.

Plato

232) What would life be if we had no courage to attempt anything?   Vincent Van Gogh

233) All life is an experiment. The more experiments you make the better.   Ralph Waldo Emerson

234) Worry is like a rocking chair: it gives you something to do but never gets you anywhere.

Erma Bombeck

235) He tried to drown his troubles but they knew how to swim.   Rita Mae Brown

236) Vitality shows in not only the ability to persist but the ability to start over.   F. Scott Fitzgerald

237) Man cannot discover new oceans unless he has the courage to lose sight of the shore.   Andre Gide

238) Those who dream by day are cognizant of many things that escape those who dream only at night.

Edgar Allan Poe

239) There are no shortcuts to any place worth going.

Beverly Sills

240) The mind ought sometimes to be diverted that it may return to better thinking.   Phaedrus

241) You can avoid reality, but you cannot avoid the consequences of avoiding reality.   Ayn Rand

242) I think I've discovered the secret of life - you just hang around until you get used to it.
                              Charles M. Schulz

243) Whatever the mind of man can conceive, it can achieve.   W. Clement Stone

244) Every calamity is to be overcome by endurance.
                                          Virgil

245) When we commit to action, to actually doing something rather than feeling trapped by events, the stress becomes manageable.   Greg Anderson

246) Don't bother just to be better than your contemporaries or predecessors. Try to be better than yourself.   William Faulkner

247) No matter how much you nurse a grudge it won't get better.   Evan Esar

248) If everything seems to be going well, you have obviously overlooked something.   Anonymous

249) Although beauty may be in the eye of the beholder, the feeling of being beautiful exists solely in the mind of the beheld.   Martha Beck

250) It is important from time to time to slow down, to go away by yourself, and simply be.   Eileen Caddy

251) There is just one life for each of us: our own.
Epictetus

252) Some people are making such thorough preparation for rainy days that they aren't enjoying today's sunshine.   William Feather

253) True friends are families which you can select.
Audrey Hepburn

254) An idea not coupled with action will never get any bigger than the brain cell it occupied.
Arnold Glasgow

255) It's being willing to walk away that gives you strength and power - if you're willing to accept the consequences of doing what you want to do.
Whoopi Goldberg

256) Each is responsible for his own actions.
H. L. Hunt

257) Believe that life is worth living and your belief will help create the fact.   William James

258) Life is a great big canvas, and you should throw all the paint on it you can.   Danny Kaye

259) Nobody got anywhere in the world by simply being content.   Louis L'Amour

260) Take life slowly and deliberately, making sure to acknowledge the people who have helped you succeed along the way.   Ted Levine

261) Money won't create success, the freedom to make it will.   Nelson Mandela

262) The advantage of having a bad memory is that, several times over, one enjoys the same good things for the first time.   Friedrich Nietzsche

263) Where belief is painful we are slow to believe.
                    Ovid

264) You have a choice. Live or die. Every breath is a choice. Every minute is a choice. To be or not to be.
                    Chuck Palahniuk

265) It is not easy to find happiness in ourselves, and it is not possible to find it elsewhere.
                    Agnes Repplier

266) The only real failure in life is the failure to try.
                    George Bernard Shaw

267) Remember, people will judge you by your actions, not your intentions. You may have a heart of gold - but so does a hard-boiled egg.   Unknown

268) The secret to a rich life is to have more beginnings than endings.   Dave Weinbaum

269) A person starts dying when they stop dreaming.
                                   Brian Williams

270) The more you praise and celebrate your life, the more there is in life to celebrate.   Oprah Winfrey

271) Eventually time takes care of everything. The trouble with procrastination is that people give up on it too soon.   Robert Brault

272) Among mortals second thoughts are wisest.
                                        Epictetus

273) Procrastination isn't the problem. It's the solution. It's the universe's way of saying stop, slow down, you move too fast.   Ellen DeGeneres

274) Aim higher in case you fall short.
                                   Suzanne Collins

275) The idea that tomorrow might get better is enough to get me through today.   Mark Amend

276) Courage is not the absence of fear, but rather the judgment that something else is more important than fear.   Meg Cabot

277) Who says life is fair, where is that written?
                                   William Goldman

278) Stop thinking of what could go wrong and start thinking of what could go right.   Harriet Morgan

279) The reason people find it so hard to be happy is that they always see the past better than it was, the present worse than it is, and the future less resolved than it will be.   Marcel Pagnol

280) Life isn't as serious as the mind makes it out to be.   Eckhart Tolle

281) They are able because they think they are able.
                    Virgil

282) Dreams come in a size too big so we can grow into them.   Josie Bisset

283) A rich man is nothing but a poor man with money.   W. C. Fields

284) Time is more valuable than money. You can get more money, but you cannot get more time.
                    Jim Rohn

285) There is no success without hardship.
                    Sophocles

286) Arguing about whether the glass is half full or half empty misses the point, which is this: the bartender cheated you.   Unknown

287) The worst part of acting like a jerk isn't when you're doing it, it's when you realize you were.
Pete Wentz

288) May all your joys be pure joys, and all your pain champagne.
Drake

289) If you've ever felt inspired by a purpose or calling, you know the feeling of spirit working through you.
Dr. Wayne W. Dyer

290) Only those who will risk going too far can possibly find out how far one can go.
T.S. Eliot

291) There isn't a person anywhere who isn't capable of doing more than he thinks he can.
Henry Ford

292) Insanity is hereditary. You get it from your kids.
Richard Gere

293) The most important thing in life is to learn how to give out love, and to let it come in.
Morrie Schwartz

294) Fear isn't an excuse to come to a standstill. It's the impetus to step up and strike.
Arthur Ashe

295) Bad things are not the worst things that can happen to us. Nothing is the worst thing that can happen to us!
Richard Bach

296) It's not the load that breaks you down, it's the way you carry it. Lou Holtz

297) If you accept the expectations of others, especially negative ones, then you never will change the outcome. Michael Jordan

298) It is better to look ahead and prepare than to look back and regret. Jackie Joyner-Kersee

299) Those who have succeeded at anything and don't mention luck are kidding themselves.
Larry King

300) You block your dream when you allow your fear to grow bigger than your faith.
Mary Manin Morrissey

301) Our mind is best prepared for gratitude when its open just as the cup is best prepared for filling when it's empty. Kemmy Nola

302) Those who think it is permissible to tell white lies soon grow color-blind. Austin O'Malley

303) Life is one grand, sweet song so start the music.
Ronald Reagan

304) A stumbling block to the pessimist is a stepping-stone to the optimist. Eleanor Roosevelt

305) Knowledge of what is possible is the beginning of happiness.   George Santayana

306) No matter what your heartache may be, laughing helps you forget it for a few seconds.
                                Red Skelton

307) Opportunity is rare, and a wise man will never let it go by him.   Bayard Taylor

308) Hearing is one of the body's five senses. But listening is an art.   Frank Tyger

309) If the left side of your brain controls the right side of your body, then only left handed people are in their right mind.   Unknown

310) Appreciation is a wonderful thing: It makes what is excellent in others belong to us as well.   Voltaire

311) Go to Heaven for the climate, Hell for the company.   Mark Twain

312) I'd rather be alone and wish I were with someone than to be with someone and wish I were alone.   Erica Allende

313) If everything is easy to get, we will never appreciate and be proud of what we have.
                                Mark Amend

314) There are no speed limits on the road to
excellence.   Richard Bach

315) A man is not old until regrets take the place of
dreams.   John Barrymore

316) The sweetest sound of all is praise.

Xenophon

317) It is not the strongest of the species that
survives, nor the most intelligent, but the one most
responsive to change.   Charles Darwin

318) Your past is always your past. Even if you forget
it, it remembers you.   Sarah Dessen

319) It isn't where you came from, its where you're
going that counts.   Ella Fitzgerald

320) Do what you're passionate about.

Lacey Chabert

321) You can never be upset with the people who
forced you into your dream or up higher.

Terry Perry

322) You don't stop laughing because you grow old.
You grow old because you stop laughing.

Michael Pritchard

323) I would much rather have regrets about not doing what people said, than regretting not doing what my heart led me to and wondering what life had been like if I'd just been myself.   Brittany Renée

324) Never give up on what you really want to do. The person with big dreams is more powerful than one with all the facts.   Unknown

www.ingramcontent.com/pod-product-compliance
Lightning Source LLC
Chambersburg PA
CBHW070653290526
45790CB00001B/305